# Nutrition
## FOR
# DUMMIES®
### PORTABLE EDITION

**by Carol Ann Rinzler**

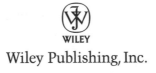

WILEY

Wiley Publishing, Inc.

# Nutrition For Dummies® Portable Edition

Published by
**Wiley Publishing, Inc.**
111 River St.
Hoboken, NJ 07030-5774
www.wiley.com

Copyright © 2010 by Wiley Publishing, Inc., Indianapolis, Indiana

Published simultaneously in Canada

For general information on our other products and services, please contact our Customer Care Department within the U.S. at 877-762-2974, outside the U.S. at 317-572-3993, or fax 317-572-4002.

For technical support, please visit www.wiley.com/techsupport.

Wiley also publishes its books in a variety of electronic formats. Some content that appears in print may not be available in electronic books.

ISBN: 978-0-470-59191-8

Manufactured in the United States of America

10  9  8  7  6  5  4  3  2  1

**Publisher's Acknowledgments**

**Editor:** Elizabeth Kuball

**Composition Services:** Indianapolis Composition Services Department

**Cover Photo:** © Thinkstock

WILEY

# Table of Contents

● ● ● ● ● ● ● ● ● ● ● ● ● ● ● ● ● ● ● ● ● ● ● ● ● ● ● ● ● ● ● ● ● ● ●

*Introduction* . . . . . . . . . . . . . . . . . . . . *1*

About This Book.................................................................1
Conventions Used in This Book......................................2
What You Don't Have to Read .......................................2
Foolish Assumptions........................................................3
Icons Used in This Book ..................................................3
Where to Go from Here....................................................4

**Chapter 1: What's Nutrition, Anyway?...............5**

Nutrition Equals Life ......................................................6
    First principles: Energy and nutrients .....................8
    What's an essential nutrient?....................................9
    Protecting the nutrients in your food .....................10
    Other interesting substances in food......................11
    You are what you eat ...............................................11
    Your nutritional status.............................................13
    Fitting food into the medicine chest ......................15
Finding Nutrition Facts .................................................15
    Nutritional people....................................................15
    Can you trust this study?.........................................17

**Chapter 2: How Much Nutrition Do You Need? . . . . . .21**

The Essentials ................................................................22
Recommendations for Carbohydrates,
    Fats, Dietary Fiber, and Alcohol............................22
Different People, Different Needs .................................24

**Chapter 3: Powerful Protein. . . . . . . . . . . . . . . . . . . . . .31**

Looking Inside and Out: Where Your
    Body Puts Protein ...................................................32
Putting Protein to Work: How Your
    Body Uses Protein...................................................32
Packing Back the Protein: What Happens
    to the Proteins You Eat ..........................................34

Examining Protein Types: Not All
  Proteins Are Created Equal .......................................35
    Essential and nonessential proteins ......................35
    High-quality and low-quality proteins...................38
    Complete proteins and incomplete proteins ........39
Deciding How Much Protein You Need ........................43
    Calculating the correct amount...............................43
    Dodging protein deficiency .....................................44
    Boosting your protein intake:
      Special considerations.........................................45
    Avoiding protein overload........................................45

**Chapter 4: The Lowdown on Fat and Cholesterol ....47**

Finding the Facts about Fat Stuff.................................48
    Understanding how your body uses fat.................48
    Pulling energy from fat.............................................49
    Focusing on the fats in food ...................................51
    Getting the right amount of fat ...............................51
    Essential fatty acids.................................................52
    Finding fat in all kinds of foods .............................53
    Defining fatty acids and their
      relationship to dietary fat...................................54
Considering Cholesterol and You ................................60
    Cholesterol and heart disease ................................60
    Living with lipoproteins...........................................63
    Diet and cholesterol .................................................65

**Chapter 5: Carbohydrates: A Complex Story.........69**

Checking Out Carbohydrates.........................................70
    Carbohydrates and energy:
      a biochemical love story .....................................72
    How glucose becomes energy..................................73
    How pasta ends up on your hips when
      too many carbs pass your lips ............................74
    Other ways your body uses carbohydrates..........75
    Finding the carbohydrates you need......................76
    Some problems with carbohydrates.......................77
    Who needs extra carbohydrates?............................77

Dietary Fiber: The Non-Nutrient in
    Carbohydrate Foods .......................................... 79
    The two kinds of dietary fiber ................................ 80
    Getting fiber from food ........................................ 81
    How much fiber do you need? ............................... 82

**Chapter 6: Water Works . . . . . . . . . . . . . . . . . . . . . . . . 87**

Investigating the Many Ways
    Your Body Uses Water .......................................... 88
Maintaining the Right Amount
    of Water in Your Body ........................................... 88
    A balancing act: The role of electrolytes ............... 89
    Dehydrating without enough water
        and electrolytes .............................................. 92
Getting the Water You Need ....................................... 93
Taking in Extra Water and Electrolytes as Needed .... 96
    You're sick to your stomach ................................. 98
    You're exercising or working hard
        in a hot environment ....................................... 99
    You're on a high-protein diet .............................. 102
    You're taking certain medications ....................... 102
    You have high blood pressure ............................. 102

**Chapter 7: What Is a Healthful Diet? . . . . . . . . . . . . 103**

What Are Dietary Guidelines for Americans? .......... 104
Controlling Your Weight ........................................... 104
    Getting the most nutritious calories ................... 104
    Managing your weight ........................................ 105
    Being physically active ....................................... 106
Making Smart Food Choices ..................................... 109
    Picking the perfect plants ................................... 109
    Figuring out fats ................................................. 110
    Counting on carbs .............................................. 111
    Limiting salt, balancing potassium .................... 111
    Moderating alcohol consumption ....................... 114
Okay, Now Relax ....................................................... 115

## Chapter 8: Making Wise Food Choices . . . . . . . . . . . .119

Playing with Blocks: Basics of the Food Pyramids... 120
    The original USDA Food Guide Pyramid.............. 120
    The brand-new 2005 USDA
        Food Guide Pyramid ......................................... 124
Understanding the Nutrition Facts Labels ................ 125
    Just the facts, ma'am............................................. 127
    Listing what's inside............................................... 132
Choosing Foods with MyPyramid and
    the Nutrition Facts Label......................................... 133
The Final Word on Diagrams and Stats ..................... 134

# Introduction

. . . . . . . . . . . . . . . . . . . . . . . . . . . . .

**O**nce upon a time, people simply sat down to
dinner, eating to fill up an empty stomach or just
for the pleasure of it. Nobody said, "Wow, that cream
soup is loaded with calories," asked whether the
bread was a high-fiber loaf, or fretted about the
chicken being served with the skin still on. No longer.
Today, the dinner table can be a battleground
between health and pleasure. You plan your meals
with the precision of a major general moving his
troops into the front lines, and for most people, the
fight to eat what's good for you rather than what
tastes good has become a lifelong struggle.

This book is designed to end the war between your
need for good nutrition and your equally compelling
need for tasty meals. In fact (listen up, here!), what's
good for you can also be good to eat — and vice versa.

## About This Book

*Nutrition For Dummies* doesn't aim to send you back to
the classroom, set you down, and make you take notes
about what to put on the table every day from now until
you're 104 years old. You're reading a reference book,
so you don't have to memorize anything — when you
want more info, just jump in anywhere to look it up.

Instead, this book means to give you the information
you need to make wise food choices — which always
means choices that please the palate and soul, as well
as the body.

*Nutrition For Dummies* includes hot new info from the 2005 revisions of the *Dietary Guidelines for Americans,* new recommended daily allowances for all the nutrients a healthy body needs, plus all the twisty "this is good for you" and "this is really, really rotten" bits and pieces of food info that nutrition scientists have come up with recently.

# Conventions Used in This Book

The following conventions are used throughout the text to make things consistent and easy to understand:

- ✔ All Web addresses appear in `monofont`.

- ✔ New terms appear in *italic* and are closely followed by an easy-to-understand definition.

- ✔ **Bold** is used to highlight the action parts of numbered steps, as well as key words in bulleted lists.

# What You Don't Have to Read

What? Not read something printed in a book? Well, yeah. Some small parts of this book are fun or informative but not necessarily vital to your understanding of nutrition. For example:

- ✔ **Text in sidebars:** The sidebars are the shaded boxes that appear here and there. They share personal stories and observations but aren't necessary reading.

- ✔ **Anything with a Technical Stuff icon attached:** This information is interesting but not critical to your understanding of nutrition.

> ✔ **The stuff on the copyright page:** No kidding.
> You'll find nothing here of interest unless you're
> inexplicably enamored by legal language and
> Library of Congress numbers.

## Foolish Assumptions

Every book is written with a particular reader in
mind, and this one is no different. As I wrote this
book, I made the following basic assumptions about
who you are and why you plunked down your hard-
earned cash for an entire volume about nutrition:

> ✔ You didn't study nutrition in high school or
> college and now you've discovered that you
> have a better shot a staying healthy if you know
> how to put together well-balanced, nutritious
> meals.
>
> ✔ You need a reliable road map through the
> nutrient maze.
>
> ✔ You want basic information, but you don't want
> to become an expert in nutrition or spend hours
> digging your way through medical textbooks
> and journals.

## Icons Used in This Book

Icons are a handy *For Dummies* way to catch your
attention as you slide your eyes down the page. The
icons come in several varieties, each with its own special meaning:

Nutrition is full of stuff that "everybody knows."
This masked marvel clues you in to the real
facts when (as often happens) everybody's
wrong!

This little guy looks smart because he's marking the place where you find definitions of the words used by nutrition experts.

 The Official Word icon says, "Look here for scientific studies, statistics, definitions, and recommendations used to create standard nutrition policy."

 This time, the same smart fella is pointing to clear, concise explanations of technical terms and processes — details that are interesting but not necessarily critical to your understanding of a topic. In other words, skip them if you want, but try a few first.

 Bull's-eye! This is time- and stress-saving information that you can use to improve your diet and health.

 This is a watch-out-for-the-curves icon, alerting you to nutrition pitfalls.

## Where to Go from Here

You've got your Portable Edition of *Nutrition For Dummies* — now what? This portable guide is a reference, so if you need information on how much fat is too much, head to Chapter 4. Or if you're interested in finding out about water, go straight to Chapter 6. Or heck, start with Chapter 1 and read the chapters in order . . . you rebel. If you want even more advice on nutrition, from the healing power of foods to how to eat smart when eating out, check out the full-size version of *Nutrition For Dummies,* 4th Edition — simply head to your local book seller or go to www.dummies.com!

# Chapter 1

# What's Nutrition, Anyway?

---

## In This Chapter

▶ Exploring why nutrition matters

▶ Determining the value of food

▶ Locating reliable sources for nutrition information

▶ Finding out how to read (and question) a nutrition study

---

*W*elcome aboard! You're about to begin your very own *Fantastic Voyage*. (You know. That's the 1966 movie in which Raquel Welch and a couple of guys were shrunk down to the size of a molecule to sail through the body of a politician shot by an assassin who had . . . hey, maybe you should just check out the next showing on your favorite cable movie channel.)

In any event, as you read, chapter by chapter, you can follow a route that carries food (meaning food and beverages) from your plate to your mouth to your digestive tract and into every tissue and cell. Along the way, you'll have the opportunity to see how your organs and systems work. You'll observe first-hand why some foods and beverages are essential to your health. And you'll discover how to manage your diet so you can get the biggest bang (nutrients) for your buck (calories). Bon voyage!

# Nutrition Equals Life

Technically speaking, *nutrition* is the science of how the body uses food. In fact, nutrition is life. All living things, including you, need food and water to live. Beyond that, you need *good* food — meaning food with the proper nutrients — to live well. If you don't eat and drink, you'll die. Period. If you don't eat and drink nutritious food and beverages:

- ✔ Your bones may bend or break (not enough calcium).

- ✔ Your gums may bleed (not enough vitamin C).

- ✔ Your blood may not carry oxygen to every cell (not enough iron).

And on, and on, and on. Understanding how good nutrition protects you against these dire consequences requires a familiarity with the language and concepts of nutrition. Knowing some basic chemistry is helpful (don't panic: Chemistry can be a cinch when you read about it in plain English). A smattering of sociology and psychology is also useful, because although nutrition is mostly about how food revs up and sustains your body, it's also about the cultural traditions and individual differences that explain how you choose your favorite foods.

To sum it up: Nutrition is about why you eat what you eat and how the food you get affects your body and your health.

# Essential nutrients for Fido, Fluffy, and your pet petunia

Vitamin C isn't the only nutrient that's essential for one species but not for others. Many *organic compounds* (substances similar to vitamins) and *elements* (minerals) are essential for your green or furry friends but not for you, either because you can synthesize them from the food you eat or because they're so widely available in the human diet and you require such small amounts that you can get what you need without hardly trying.

Two good examples are the organic compounds choline and myoinositol. *Choline* is an essential nutrient for several species of animals, including dogs, cats, rats, and guinea pigs. Although choline is essential for human beings, human bodies produce choline on their own, and you can get choline from eggs, liver, soybeans, cauliflower, and lettuce. *Myoinositol* is an essential nutrient for gerbils and rats, but human beings synthesize it naturally and use it in many body processes, such as transmitting signals between cells.

Here's a handy list of nutrients that are essential for animals and/or plants but not for you:

| Organic Compounds | Elements |
|---|---|
| Carnitine | Arsenic |
| Myoinositol | Cadmium |
| Taurine | Lead |
|  | Nickel |
|  | Silicon |
|  | Tin |
|  | Vanadium |

## *First principles: Energy and nutrients*

Nutrition's primary task is figuring out which foods and beverages (in what quantities) provide the energy and building material you need to construct and maintain every organ and system. To do this, nutrition concentrates on food's two basic attributes: energy and nutrients.

*Energy* is the ability to do work. Virtually every bite of food gives you energy, even when it doesn't give you nutrients. The amount of energy in food is measured in *calories,* the amount of heat produced when food is burned (metabolized) in your body cells. Food is the fuel on which your body runs. Without enough food, you don't have enough energy.

*Nutrients* are chemical substances that your body uses to build, maintain, and repair tissues. They also empower cells to send messages back and forth to conduct essential chemical reactions, such as the ones that make it possible for you to

- ✔ Breathe
- ✔ Move
- ✔ Eliminate waste
- ✔ Think
- ✔ See
- ✔ Hear
- ✔ Smell
- ✔ Taste

. . . and do everything else natural to a living body.

Food provides two distinct groups of nutrients:

- **Macronutrients (*macro* = big):** Protein, fat, carbohydrates, and water
- **Micronutrients (*micro* = small):** Vitamins and minerals

What's the difference between these two groups? The amount you need each day. Your daily requirements for macronutrients generally exceed 1 gram. (For comparison's sake, 28 grams are in an ounce.) For example, a man needs about 63 grams of protein a day (slightly more than 2 ounces), and a woman needs 50 grams (slightly less than 2 ounces).

Your daily requirements for micronutrients are much smaller. For example, the Recommended Dietary Allowance (RDA) for vitamin C is measured in *milligrams* (1/1,000 of a gram), while the RDAs for vitamin D, vitamin B12, and folate are even smaller and are measured in *micrograms* (1/1,000,000 of a gram). You can find out much more about the RDAs, including how they vary for people of different ages, in Chapter 2.

## What's an essential nutrient?

A reasonable person may assume that an essential nutrient is one you need to sustain a healthy body. But who says a reasonable person thinks like a nutritionist? In nutritionspeak, an *essential nutrient* is a very special thing:

- **An essential nutrient cannot be manufactured in the body.** You have to get essential nutrients from food or from a nutritional supplement.

✔ **An essential nutrient is linked to a specific deficiency disease.** For example, people who go without protein for extended periods of time develop
the protein-deficiency disease *kwashiorkor*. People
who don't get enough vitamin C develop the
vitamin C–deficiency disease *scurvy*. A diet rich
in the essential nutrient cures the deficiency
disease, but you need the proper nutrient. In
other words, you can't cure a protein deficiency
with extra amounts of vitamin C.

Not all nutrients are essential for all species of animals. For example, vitamin C is an essential nutrient
for human beings but not for dogs. A dog's body
makes the vitamin C it needs. Check out the list of
nutrients on a can or bag of dog food. See? No C. The
dog already has the C he requires.

Essential nutrients for human beings include many
well-known vitamins and minerals, several *amino
acids* (the so-called building blocks of proteins), and
at least two fatty acids.

## Protecting the nutrients in your food

Identifying nutrients is one thing. Making sure you get
them into your body is another. Here, the essential
idea is to keep nutritious food nutritious by preserv-
ing and protecting its components.

Some people see the term *food processing* as a nutritional dirty word (or words). They're wrong. Without
food processing and preservatives, you and I would
still be forced to gather (or kill) our food each morning and down it fast before it spoiled.

Considering how vital food preservation can be, you
may want to think about when you last heard a rous-
ing cheer for the anonymous cook who first noticed

that salting or pickling food could extend food's shelf life. Or for the guys who invented the refrigeration and freezing techniques that slow food's natural tendency to degrade (translation: spoil). Or for Louis Pasteur, the man who made it ab-so-lute-ly clear that heating food to boiling kills bugs that might otherwise cause food poisoning. Hardly ever, that's when. So give them a hand, right here. Cool.

## *Other interesting substances in food*

The latest flash in the nutrition sky is caused by phytochemicals. *Phyto* is the Greek word for plants, so *phytochemicals* are simply — yes, you've got it — chemicals from plants. Although the 13-letter group name may be new to you, you're already familiar with some phytochemicals. Vitamins are phytochemicals. Pigments such as beta carotene — the deep yellow coloring in fruits and vegetables that your body can convert to a form of vitamin A — are phytochemicals.

And then there are *phytoestrogens,* hormone-like chemicals that grabbed the spotlight when it was suggested that a diet high in phytoestrogens, such as the isoflavones found in soybeans, may lower the risk of heart disease and reduce the incidence of reproductive cancers (cancers of the breast, ovary, uterus, and prostate). More recent studies suggest that phytoestrogens may have some problems of their own. (To find out more about phytochemicals, including phytoestrogens, check out the full-size version of *Nutrition For Dummies,* 4th Edition.)

## *You are what you eat*

Oh boy, I bet you've heard this one before. But it bears repeating, because the human body really is built from the nutrients it gets from food: water, protein, fat, carbohydrates, vitamins, and minerals. On average, when you step on the scale

- ✔ About 60 percent of your weight is water.
- ✔ About 20 percent of your weight is fat.
- ✔ About 20 percent of your weight is a combination of mostly protein (especially in your muscles) plus carbohydrates, minerals, and vitamins.

 An easy way to remember your body's percentage of water, fat, and protein and other nutrients is to think of it as the "60-20-20 Rule."

---

## What's a body made of?

Sugar and spice and everything nice. . . . Oops. What I meant to say was the human body is made of water and fat and protein and carbohydrates and vitamins and minerals.

On average, when you step on the scale, approximately 60 percent of your weight is water, 20 percent is body fat (slightly less for a man), and 20 percent is a combination of mostly protein, plus carbohydrates, minerals, vitamins, and other naturally occurring biochemicals.

Based on these percentages, you can reasonably expect that an average 140-pound person's body weight consists of about

- ✔ 84 pounds of water
- ✔ 28 pounds of body fat
- ✔ 28 pounds of a combination of protein (up to 25 pounds), minerals (up to 7 pounds), carbohydrates (up to 1.4 pounds), and vitamins (a trace)

Yep, you're right: Those last figures do total more than 28 pounds. That's because "up to" (as in "up to 25 pounds of protein") means that the amounts may vary from person to person.

For example, a young person's body has proportionately more muscle and less fat than an older person's, while a woman's body has proportionately less muscle and more fat than a man's. As a result, more of a man's weight comes from protein and calcium, while more of a woman's body comes from fat. Protein-packed muscles and mineral-packed bones are denser tissue than fat.

Weigh a man and a woman of roughly the same height and size, and he's likely to tip the scale higher every time.

Source: The National Research Council, *Recommended Dietary Allowances* (Washington D.C.: National Academy Press, 1989); Eleanor Noss Whitney, Corinne Balog Cataldo, and Sharon Rady Rolfes, *Understanding Normal and Clinical Nutrition* (Minneapolis/St. Paul: West Publishing Company, 1994)

## *Your nutritional status*

*Nutritional status* is a phrase that describes the state of your health as related to your diet. For example, people who are starving do not get the nutrients or calories they need for optimum health. These people are said to be *malnourished* (*mal* = bad), which means that their nutritional status is, to put it gently, definitely not good.

Malnutrition may arise from

 ✔ **A diet that doesn't provide enough food:** This situation can occur in times of famine or through voluntary starvation because of an eating disorder or because something in your life disturbs your appetite. For example, older people may be at risk of malnutrition because of tooth loss or age-related loss of appetite or because they live alone and sometimes just forget to eat.

✔ **A diet that, while otherwise adequate, is deficient in a specific nutrient:** This kind of nutritional inadequacy can lead to a deficiency disease, such as beriberi, the disease caused by a lack of vitamin B1.

✔ **A metabolic disorder or medical condition that prevents your body from absorbing specific nutrients, such as carbohydrates or protein.** One common example is diabetes, the inability to produce enough *insulin,* the hormone your body uses to digest carbohydrates. Another is celiac disease, a condition that makes it impossible for the body to digest gluten, a protein in wheat. (Need more info on either diabetes or celiac disease? Check out *Diabetes For Dummies,* 3rd Edition, by Alan L. Rubin, MD, and *Living Gluten-Free For Dummies,* by Danna Korn, both published by Wiley.)

Doctors and registered dieticians have many tools with which to rate your nutritional status. For example, they can

✔ Review your medical history to see whether you have any conditions (such as dentures) that may make eating certain foods difficult or that interfere with your ability to absorb nutrients.

✔ Perform a physical examination to look for obvious signs of nutritional deficiency, such as dull hair and eyes, poor posture, or extreme thinness.

✔ Order laboratory blood and urine tests that may identify early signs of malnutrition, such as the lack of red blood cells that characterizes anemia caused by an iron deficiency.

*Remember:* At every stage of life, the aim of a good diet is to maintain a healthy nutritional status.

## Fitting food into the medicine chest

Food is medicine for the body and the soul. Good meals make good friends, and modern research validates the virtues of not only Granny's chicken soup but also heart-healthy sulfur compounds in garlic and onions, anti-cholesterol dietary fiber in grains and beans, bone-building calcium in milk and greens, and mood elevators in coffee, tea, and chocolate.

Of course, foods pose some risks as well: food allergies, food intolerances, food and drug interactions, and the occasional harmful substances such as the dreaded *saturated fats* and *trans fats* (quick — Chapter 4!). In other words, constructing a healthful diet can mean tailoring food choices to your own special body. Not to worry: You can do it. Especially after reading through Chapters 7 and 8. Would a *For Dummies* book leave you unarmed? Not a chance!

# Finding Nutrition Facts

Getting reliable information about nutrition can be a daunting challenge. For the most part, your nutrition information is likely to come from TV and radio talk shows or news, your daily newspaper, your favorite magazine, a variety of nutrition-oriented books, and the Internet. How can you tell whether what you hear or read is really right?

## Nutritional people

The people who make nutrition news may be scientists, reporters, or simply someone who wandered in with a new theory (Artichokes prevent cancer! Never eat cherries and cheese at the same meal! Vitamin C gives you hives!), the more bizarre the better. But several groups of people are most likely to give you news you can use with confidence. For example:

- **Nutrition scientists:** These are people with graduate degrees (usually in chemistry, biology, biochemistry, or physics) engaged in research dealing primarily with the effects of food on animals and human beings.

- **Nutrition researchers:** Researchers may be either nutrition scientists or professionals in another field, such as medicine or sociology, whose research concentrates on the effects of food.

- **Nutritionists:** These are people who concentrate on the study of nutrition. In some states, a person who uses the title "nutritionist" must have a graduate degree in basic science courses related to nutrition.

- **Dietitians:** These people have undergraduate degrees in food and nutrition science or the management of food programs. A person with the letters RD after his name has completed a dietetic internship and passed an American Dietetic Association licensing exam.

- **Nutrition reporters and writers:** These people specialize in giving you information about the medical and/or scientific aspects of food. Like reporters who concentrate on politics or sports, nutrition reporters gain their expertise through years of covering their beat. Most have the science background required to translate technical information into language nonscientists can understand; some have been trained as dietitians, nutritionists, or nutrition scientists.

Consumer alert: Regardless of the source, nutrition news should always pass what you may call *The Reasonableness Test*. In other words, if a story or report or study sounds ridiculous, it probably is.

Want some guidelines for evaluating nutrition studies? Read on.

## Can you trust this study?

You open your morning newspaper or turn on the evening news and read or hear that a group of researchers at an impeccably prestigious scientific organization has published a study showing that yet another thing you've always taken for granted is hazardous to your health. For example, the study says drinking coffee stresses your heart, adding salt to food raises blood pressure, or fatty foods increase your risk of cancer or heart disease.

So you throw out the offending food or drink or rearrange your daily routine to avoid the once-acceptable, now-dangerous food, beverage, or additive. And then what happens? Two weeks, two months, or two years down the road, a second, equally prestigious group of scientists publishes a study conclusively proving that the first group got it wrong: In fact, this study shows coffee has no effect on the risk of heart disease — and may even improve athletic performance; salt does not cause hypertension except in certain sensitive individuals; only *some* fatty foods are risky.

Who's right? Nobody seems to know. That leaves you, a layperson, on your own to come up with the answer. Never fear — you may not be a nutritionist, but that doesn't mean you can't apply a few common-sense rules to any study you read about, rules that say: "Yes, this may be true," or "No, this may not be."

Start by asking whether the study includes human beings. True, animal studies can alert researchers to potential problems, but working with animals alone cannot give you conclusive proof.

Different species react differently to various chemicals and diseases. For example, although cows and horses can digest grass and hay, human being can't. And although outright poisons such as cyanide clearly traumatize any living body, many foods or drugs that harm a laboratory rat won't harm you. And vice versa.

For example, mouse and rat embryos suffer no ill effects when their mothers are given thalidomide, the sedative that's known to cause deformed fetal limbs when given to pregnant monkeys — and human beings — at the point in pregnancy when limbs are developing.

And here's an astounding turn: Modern research shows that thalidomide is beneficial for treating or preventing *human* skin problems related to Hansen's disease (leprosy), cancer, and/or autoimmune conditions, such as rheumatoid arthritis, in which the body mistakenly attacks its own tissues.

Another key question to ask is: Are enough people in this study? Hey, researchers' saying, "Well, I did give this to a couple of people," is simply not enough. The study must include sufficient numbers and a variety of individuals, too. If you don't have enough people in the study — several hundred to many thousand — to establish a pattern, there's always the possibility that an effect occurred by chance.

If you don't include different types of people, which generally means young and old men and women of different racial and ethnic groups, your results may not apply across the board. For example, the original studies linking high blood cholesterol levels to an increased risk of heart disease and linking small doses of aspirin to a reduced risk of a second heart attack involved only men. It wasn't until follow-up studies were conducted with women that researchers were able to say with any certainty that high cholesterol is dangerous and aspirin is protective for women as well — but not in quite the same way: In January 2006, the *Journal of the American Medical Association* reported that men taking low-dose aspirin tend to lower their risk of heart attack. For women, the aspirin reduces the risk of stroke.

 Also consider: Might anything in the design or method of this study affect the accuracy of its conclusions? Some testing methods are more likely to lead to biased or inaccurate conclusions. For example, a *retrospective study* (which asks people to tell what they did in the past) is always considered less accurate than a *prospective study* (one that follows people while they're actually doing what the researchers are studying), because memory isn't always accurate. People tend to forget details or unintentionally alter them to fit the researchers' questions.

 Finally, ask yourself: Are the study's conclusions reasonable? When a study comes up with a conclusion that seems illogical to you, chances are, the researchers feel the same way.

For example, in 1990, the long-running Nurses' Study at the Harvard School of Public Health reported that a high-fat diet raised the risk of colon cancer. But the data showed a link only to diets high in beef. No link was found to diets high in dairy fat. In short, this study was begging for a second study to confirm (or deny) its results.

And while we wait for that second and, naturally, third study, you can bet we're keeping an open mind. The nature of life is that things *do* change, sometimes in surprising ways. Consider dioxin, a toxic contaminant found in some fish. Consider Olestra, the calorie-free fat substitute that makes some tummies rumble. As you read this page, dioxin's still a bad actor, but in 2005 researchers at the University of Cincinnati and the University of Western Australia announced that eating foods containing Olestra may speed your body's elimination of — you guessed it — dioxin. Amazing.

# Chapter 2

# How Much Nutrition Do You Need?

. . . . . . . . . . . . . . . . . . . . . . . . . . . . . . . .

## In This Chapter

▶ Unveiling the Recommended Dietary Allowances

▶ Discovering how who you are determines the amount of nutrients you need

. . . . . . . . . . . . . . . . . . . . . . . . . . . . . . . .

A healthful diet provides sufficient amounts of all the nutrients that your body needs. The question is, how much is enough?

The most familiar set of recommendations, and the one I focus on here, is the Recommended Dietary Allowances (RDAs). (For information on the other two sets of recommendations— Adequate Intake [AI] and Dietary Reference Intake [DRI], see the full-size version of *Nutrition For Dummies,* 4th Edition.)

RDAs originally were designed to make planning several days' meals in advance easy for you. The *D* in RDA stands for dietary, not daily, because the RDAs are an average. You may get more of a nutrient one day and less the next, but the idea is to hit an average over several days.

In this chapter, I tell you everything you need to know about the RDAs.

# The Essentials

RDAs offer recommendations for protein and 18 essential vitamins and minerals, which include:

| | |
|---|---|
| Copper | Folate |
| Iodine | Iron |
| Magnesium | Niacin |
| Phosphorus | Selenium |
| Vitamin A | Vitamin B1 (Thiamin) |
| Vitamin B2 (Riboflavin) | Vitamin B6 |
| Vitamin B12 | Vitamin C |
| Vitamin D | Vitamin E |
| Vitamin K | Zinc |

The newest essential nutrient, choline, won its wings in 2002, but no RDAs have yet been established.

# Recommendations for Carbohydrates, Fats, Dietary Fiber, and Alcohol

What nutrients are missing from the RDA list of essentials? Carbohydrates, fiber, fat, and alcohol. The reason is simple: If your diet provides enough protein, vitamins, and minerals, it's almost certain to provide enough carbohydrates and probably more than enough fat. Although no specific RDAs exist for carbohydrates and fat, guidelines definitely exist for them and for dietary fiber and alcohol.

In 1980, the U.S. Public Health Service and the U.S. Department of Agriculture joined forces to produce the first edition of *Dietary Guidelines for Americans* (see Chapter 7). This report has been modified many times. The latest set of recommendations, issued in the spring of 2005, sets parameters for what you can consider reasonable amounts of calories, carbohydrates, dietary fiber, fats, protein, and alcohol. According to these guidelines, as a general rule, you need to

✔ **Balance your calorie intake with energy output in the form of regular exercise.**

✔ **Eat enough carbohydrates (primarily the complex ones from fruits, vegetables, and whole grains) to account for 45 to 65 percent of your total daily calories.** That's 900 to 1,300 calories on a 2,000-calorie diet.

✔ **Take in an appropriate amount of dietary fiber, currently described as 14 grams dietary fiber for every 1,000 calories.**

✔ **Get no more than 20 to 35 percent of your daily calories from dietary fat.** Therefore, if your daily diet includes about 2,000 calories, only 400 to 700 calories should come from fat. Less than 10 percent of your daily calories should come from saturated fatty acids, and your daily diet should have less than 300 milligrams cholesterol.

Eat as little trans fat as possible. The Nutrition Facts label on foods now shows a gram amount for trans fats, but there's no upper limit because any amount is considered, well, less than okey-dokey. (For the skinny on saturated, unsaturated, and trans fats, plus cholesterol, check out Chapter 4.)

✔ **Drink alcoholic beverages in moderation (if you choose to drink at all).** What's moderation? One drink a day for a woman, two for a man.

# Different People, Different Needs

Because different bodies require different amounts of nutrients, RDAs currently address as many as 22 specific categories of human beings: boys and girls, men and women, from infancy through middle age.

But who you are affects the recommendations. If age is important, so is gender. For example, because women of childbearing age lose iron when they menstruate, their RDA for iron is higher than the RDA for men. On the other hand, because men who are sexually active lose zinc through their ejaculations, the zinc RDA for men is higher than the zinc RDA for women.

Finally, gender affects body composition, which influences RDAs. Consider protein: The RDA for protein is set in terms of grams of protein per kilogram (2.2 pounds) of body weight. Because the average man weighs more than the average woman, his RDA for protein is higher than hers. The RDA for an adult male, age 19 or older, is 56 grams; for a woman, it's 46 grams.

Table 2-1 shows the most recent RDAs for vitamins for healthy adults; Table 2-2 shows RDAs for minerals for healthy adults. Where no RDA is given, an AI is indicated by an asterisk (*) by the column heading. The complete reports on which this table is based are available online. Go to www.iom.edu/Object. File/Master/21/372/0.pdf.

*Note:* In Table 2-1, I use the following abbreviations: g = gram, mg = milligram, mcg = microgram, RE = retinol equivalent, a-TE = alpha-tocopherol equivalent, and NE = niacin equivalent.

| Table 2-1 | | | | | | | Vitamin RDAs for Healthy Adults | | | | | | | | |
|---|---|---|---|---|---|---|---|---|---|---|---|---|---|---|---|
| Age (Years) | Vita- min A (RE/ IU)† | Vita- min D (mcg/ IU)‡* | Vita- min E (a-TE) | Vita- min K (mcg)* | Vita- min C (mg) | Thiamin (Vita- min B1) (mg) | Ribo- flavin (Vitamin B2) (mg) | Nia- cin (NE) | Panto- thenic acid (mg)* | Vita- min B6 (mg) | Folate (mcg) | Vita- min B12 (mcg) | Biotin (mcg)* |
| **Males** | | | | | | | | | | | | | |
| 19–30 | 900/ 2,970 | 5/200 | 15 | 120 | 90 | 1.2 | 1.3 | 16 | 5 | 1.3 | 400 | 2.4 | 30 |
| 31–50 | 900/ 2,970 | 5/200 | 15 | 120 | 90 | 1.2 | 1.3 | 16 | 5 | 1.3 | 400 | 2.4 | 30 |
| 51–70 | 900/ 2,970 | 10/400 | 15 | 120 | 90 | 1.2 | 1.3 | 16 | 5 | 1.7 | 400 | 2.4 | 30 |
| Older than 70 | 900/ 2,970 | 15/600 | 15 | 120 | 90 | 1.2 | 1.1 | 16 | 5 | 1.7 | 400 | 2.4 | 30 |

*(continued)*

**Table 2-1 (continued)**

| Age (Years) | Vita-min A (RE/IU)† | Vita-min D (mcg/IU)‡* | Vita-min E (a-TE) | Vita-min K (mcg)* | Vita-min C (mg) | Thiamin (Vita-min B1) (mg) | Ribo-flavin (Vitamin B2) (mg) | Nia-cin (NE) | Panto-thenic acid (mg)* | Vita-min B6 (mg) | Folate (mcg) | Vita-min B12 (mcg) | Biotin (mcg)* |
|---|---|---|---|---|---|---|---|---|---|---|---|---|---|
| **Females** | | | | | | | | | | | | | |
| 19–30 | 700/2,310 | 5/200 | 15 | 90 | 75 | 1.1 | 1.1 | 14 | 5 | 1.3 | 400 | 2.4 | 30 |
| 31–50 | 700/2,310 | 5/200 | 15 | 90 | 75 | 1.1 | 1.1 | 14 | 5 | 1.3 | 400 | 2.4 | 30 |
| 51–70 | 700/2,310 | 10/400 | 15 | 90 | 75 | 1.1 | 1.1 | 14 | 5 | 1.5 | 400 | 2.4 | 30 |
| Older than 70 | 700/2,310 | 15/600 | 15 | 90 | 75 | 1.1 | 1.1 | 14 | 5 | 1.5 | 400 | 2.4 | 30 |

| Age (Years) | Vita-min A (RE/IU)† | Vita-min D (mcg/IU)‡* | Vita-min E (a-TE) | Vita-min K (mcg)* | Vita-min C (mg) | Thiamin (Vita-min B1) (mg) | Ribo-flavin (Vitamin B2) (mg) | Nia-cin (NE) | Panto-thenic acid (mg)* | Vita-min B6 (mg) | Folate (mcg) | Vita-min B12 (mcg) | Biotin (mcg)* |
|---|---|---|---|---|---|---|---|---|---|---|---|---|---|
| Pregnant (age-based) | 750–770/ 2,475–2,541 | 5/200 | 15 | 75–90 | 70 | 1.4 | 1.1 | 18 | 6 | 1.9 | 600 | 2.6 | 30 |
| Nursing (age-based) | 1,200–1,300/ 3,960–4,290 | 5/200 | 19 | 76–90 | 95 | 1.4 | 1.1 | 17 | 7 | 2.0 | 500 | 2.8 | 35 |

* Adequate Intake (AI)

† The "official" RDA for vitamin A is still 1,000 RE/5,000 IU for a male, 800 RE/4,000 IU for a female who isn't pregnant or nursing; the lower numbers listed on this chart are the currently recommended levels for adults.

‡ The current recommendations are the amounts required to prevent vitamin D deficiency disease; recent studies suggest that the optimal levels for overall health may actually be higher, in the range of 800 to 1,000 IU a day.

**Table 2-2    Mineral RDAs for Healthy Adults**

| Age (years) | Cal-cium (mg)* | Phos-phorus (mg) | Mag-nesium (mg) | Iron (mg) | Zinc (mg) | Copper (mcg) | Iodine (mcg) | Sele-nium (mcg) | Molyb-denum (mcg) | Man-ganese (mg)* | Fluo-ride (mg)* | Chro-mium (mcg)* | Cho-line (mg)* |
|---|---|---|---|---|---|---|---|---|---|---|---|---|---|
| **Males** | | | | | | | | | | | | | |
| 19–30 | 1,000 | 700 | 400 | 8 | 11 | 900 | 150 | 55 | 45 | 2.3 | 4 | 36 | 550 |
| 31–50 | 1,000 | 700 | 420 | 8 | 11 | 900 | 150 | 55 | 45 | 2.3 | 4 | 36 | 550 |
| 51–70 | 1,200 | 700 | 420 | 8 | 11 | 900 | 150 | 55 | 45 | 2.3 | 4 | 30 | 550 |
| Older than 70 | 1,200 | 700 | 420 | 8 | 11 | 900 | 150 | 55 | 45 | 2.3 | 4 | 30 | 550 |
| **Females** | | | | | | | | | | | | | |
| 19–30 | 1,000 | 700 | 310 | 18 | 8 | 900 | 150 | 55 | 45 | 1.8 | 3 | 25 | 425 |
| 31–50 | 1,000 | 700 | 320 | 18 | 8 | 900 | 150 | 55 | 45 | 1.8 | 3 | 25 | 425 |
| 51–70 | 1,000/1,500** | 700 | 320 | 8 | 8 | 900 | 150 | 55 | 45 | 1.8 | 3 | 20 | 425 |

| Age (years) | Cal-cium (mg)* | Phos-phorus (mg) | Mag-nesium (mg) | Iron (mg) | Zinc (mg) | Copper (mcg) | Iodine (mcg) | Sele-nium (mcg) | Molyb-denum (mcg) | Man-ganese (mg)* | Fluo-ride (mg)* | Chro-mium (mcg)* | Cho-line (mg)* |
|---|---|---|---|---|---|---|---|---|---|---|---|---|---|
| Older than 70 | 1,000/1,500** | 700 | 320 | 8 | 8 | 900 | 150 | 55 | 45 | 1.8 | 3 | 20 | 425 |
| Pregnant | 1,000–1,300 | 700–1,250 | 350–400 | 27 | 11–12 | 1,000 | 220 | 60 | 50 | 2.0 | 1.5–4.0 | 29–30 | 450 |
| Nursing | 1,000–1,300 | 700–1,250 | 310–350 | 9–10 | 12–13 | 1,300 | 290 | 70 | 50 | 2.6 | 1.5–4.0 | 44–45 | 550 |

* Adequate Intake (AI)

** The lower recommendation is for postmenopausal women taking estrogen supplements; the higher figure is for postmenopausal women not taking estrogen supplements.

Source: Adapted with permission from Recommended Dietary Allowances (Washington D.C.: National Academy Press, 1989), and DRI panel reports, 1997–2004

# Reviewing terms used to describe nutrient recommendations

Nutrient listings use the metric system. RDAs for protein are listed in grams. The RDA for vitamins and minerals are shown in milligrams (mg) and micrograms (mcg). A milligram is 1/100 of a gram; a microgram is 1/100 of a milligram.

Vitamin A, vitamin D, and vitamin E are special cases. For instance, one form of vitamin A is *preformed vitamin A,* a form of the nutrient that your body can use right away. Preformed vitamin A, known as *retinol,* is found in food from animals — liver, milk, and eggs. Carotenoids (red or yellow pigments in plants) also provide vitamin A. But to get vitamin A from carotenoids, your body has to convert the pigments to chemicals similar to retinol. Because retinol is a ready-made nutrient, the RDA for vitamin A is listed in units called retinol equivalents (RE). One mcg (microgram) RE is approximately equal to 3.33 international units (IU, the former unit of measurement for vitamin A).

Vitamin D consists of three compounds: vitamin D1, vitamin D2, and vitamin D3. Cholecalciferol, the chemical name for vitamin D3, is the most active of the three, so the RDA for vitamin D is measured in equivalents of cholecalciferol.

Your body gets vitamin E from two classes of chemicals in food: tocopherols and tocotrienols. The compound with the greatest vitamin E activity is a tocopherol: *alpha*-tocopherol. The RDA for vitamin E is measured in milligrams of *alpha*-tocopherol equivalents (a-TE).

# Chapter 3

# Powerful Protein

· · · · · · · · · · · · · · · · · · · · · · · · · · · · · · · ·

*In This Chapter*

▶ Determining what protein is

▶ Finding the proteins in your body

▶ Getting the best-quality protein from food

▶ Gauging how much protein you need

· · · · · · · · · · · · · · · · · · · · · · · · · · · · · · · ·

*P*rotein is an essential nutrient whose name comes from the Greek word *protos,* which means "first." To visualize a molecule of protein, close your eyes and see a very long chain, rather like a chain of sausage links. The links in the chains are *amino acids,* commonly known as the building blocks of protein. In addition to carbon, hydrogen, and oxygen atoms, amino acids contain a nitrogen (amino) group. The *amino group* is essential for synthesizing (assembling) specialized proteins in your body.

In this chapter, you can find out more — maybe even more than you ever wanted to know — about this molecule, how your body uses the proteins you take in as food, and how the body makes some special proteins you need for a healthy life.

# Looking Inside and Out: Where Your Body Puts Protein

The human body is chock-full of proteins. Proteins are present in the outer and inner membranes of every living cell. Here's where else protein makes an appearance:

✔ Your hair, your nails, and the outer layers of your skin are made of the protein keratin. Keratin is a *scleroprotein*, or a protein resistant to digestive enzymes. So if you bite your nails, you can't digest them.

✔ Muscle tissue contains myosin, actin, myoglobin, and a number of other proteins.

✔ Bone has plenty of protein. The outer part of bone is hardened with minerals such as calcium, but the basic, rubbery inner structure is protein; and bone marrow, the soft material inside the bone, also contains protein.

✔ Red blood cells contain *hemoglobin*, a protein compound that carries oxygen throughout the body. *Plasma*, the clear fluid in blood, contains fat and protein particles known as *lipoproteins*, which ferry cholesterol around and out of the body.

# Putting Protein to Work: How Your Body Uses Protein

Your body uses proteins to build new cells, maintain tissues, and synthesize new proteins that make it possible for you to perform basic bodily functions.

About half the dietary protein that you consume each day goes into making *enzymes*, the specialized worker proteins that do specific jobs such as digesting food and assembling or dividing molecules to make new cells and chemical substances. To perform these functions, enzymes often need specific vitamins and minerals.

# DNA/RNA

*Nucleoproteins* are chemicals in the nucleus of every living cell. They're made of proteins linked to *nucleic acids* — complex compounds that contain phosphoric acid, a sugar molecule, and nitrogen-containing molecules made from amino acids.

Nucleic acids (molecules found in the chromosomes and other structures in the center of your cells) carry the genetic codes — genes that help determine what you look like, your general intelligence, and who you are. They contain one of two sugars, either *ribose* or *deoxyribose.* The nucleic acid containing ribose is called *ribonucleic acid* (RNA). The nucleic acid containing deoxyribose is called *deoxyribonucleic acid* (DNA).

DNA, a long molecule with two strands twisting about each other (the *double helix*), carries and transmits the genetic inheritance in your chromosomes. In other words, DNA supplies instructions that determine how your body cells are formed and how they behave. RNA, a single-strand molecule, is created in the cell nucleus according to the pattern determined by the DNA. Then RNA carries the DNA's instructions to the rest of the cell.

Knowing about DNA is important because it's the most distinctly "you" thing about your body. Chances that another person on Earth has exactly the same DNA as you are really small. That's why DNA analysis is used increasingly in identifying criminals or exonerating the innocent. Some people are even proposing that parents store a sample of their children's DNA so that they'll have a conclusive way of identifying a missing child, even years later.

Your ability to see, think, hear, and move — in fact, to do just about everything that you consider part of a healthy life — requires your nerve cells to send messages back and forth to each other and to other specialized kinds of cells, such as muscle cells. Sending these messages requires chemicals called *neurotransmitters*. Making neurotransmitters requires — guess what — proteins.

Finally, proteins play an important part in the creation of every new cell and every new individual. Your chromosomes consist of *nucleoproteins*, which are substances made of amino acids and nucleic acids.

# *Packing Back the Protein: What Happens to the Proteins You Eat*

The cells in your digestive tract can absorb only single amino acids or very small chains of two or three amino acids called *peptides*. So proteins from food are broken into their component amino acids by digestive enzymes — which are, of course, specialized proteins. Then other enzymes in your body cells build new proteins by reassembling the amino acids into specific compounds that your body needs to function. This process is called *protein synthesis*.

During protein synthesis

🗸 Amino acids hook up with fats to form *lipoproteins,* the molecules that ferry cholesterol around and out of the body. Or amino acids may join up with carbohydrates to form the *glycoproteins* found in the mucus secreted by the digestive tract.

🗸 Proteins combine with phosphoric acid to produce *phosphoproteins,* such as casein, a protein in milk.

> ✔ Nucleic acids combine with proteins to create
> *nucleoproteins,* which are essential components
> of the cell nucleus and of cytoplasm, the living
> material inside each cell.

The carbon, hydrogen, and oxygen that are left over
after protein synthesis is complete are converted to
glucose and used for energy. The nitrogen residue
(ammonia) isn't used for energy. It's processed by the
liver, which converts the ammonia to urea. Most of
the urea produced in the liver is excreted through the
kidneys in urine; very small amounts are sloughed off
in skin, hair, and nails.

Every day, you *turn over* (reuse) more proteins than
you get from the food you eat, so you need a continu-
ous supply to maintain your protein status. If your
diet does not contain sufficient amounts of proteins,
you start digesting the proteins in your body, including the proteins in your muscles and — in extreme
cases — your heart muscle.

# Examining Protein Types: Not All Proteins Are Created Equal

All proteins are made of building blocks called amino
acids, but not all proteins contain all the amino acids
you require. This section helps you figure out how
you can get the most useful proteins from your varied
diet.

## Essential and nonessential proteins

To make all the proteins that your body needs, you
require 22 different amino acids. Ten are considered
*essential,* which means you can't synthesize them in
your body and must obtain them from food (two of

these, arginine and histidine, are essential only for
children). Several more are *nonessential:* If you don't
get them in food, you can manufacture them yourself
from fats, carbohydrates, and other amino acids.
Three — glutamine, ornithine, and taurine — are
somewhere in between essential and nonessential for
human beings: They're essential only under certain
conditions, such as with injury or disease.

| Essential Amino Acids | Nonessential Amino Acids |
|---|---|
| Arginine* | Alanine |
| Histidine* | Asparagine |
| Isoleucine | Aspartic acid |
| Leucine | Citrulline |
| Lysine | Cysteine |
| Methionine | Glutamic acid |
| Phenlyalanine | Glycine |
| Threonine | Hydroxyglutamic acid |
| Tryptophan | Norleucine |
| Valine | Proline |
| | Serine |
| | Tyrosine |

* Essential for children; nonessential for adults

## Super soy: The special protein food

**Nutrition fact no. 1:** Food from animals has complete proteins. **Nutrition fact no. 2:** Vegetables, fruits, and grains have incomplete proteins. **Nutrition fact no. 3:** Nobody told the soybean.

Unlike other vegetables, including other beans, soybeans have complete proteins with sufficient amounts of all the amino acids essential to human health. In fact, food experts rank soy proteins on par with egg whites and casein (the protein in milk), the two proteins easiest for your body to absorb and use.

Some nutritionists think soy proteins are even better than the proteins in eggs and milk, because the proteins in soy come with no cholesterol and very little of the saturated fat known to clog your arteries and raise your risk of heart attack. Better yet, more than 20 recent studies suggest that adding soy foods to your diet can actually lower your cholesterol levels.

One-half cup of cooked soybeans has 14 grams of protein; 4 ounces of tofu has 13. Either serving gives you approximately twice the protein you get from one large egg or one 8-ounce glass of skim milk, or two-thirds the protein in 3 ounces of lean ground beef. Eight ounces of fat-free soy milk has 7 milligrams protein — a mere 1 milligram less than a similar serving of skim milk — and no cholesterol. Soybeans are also jam-packed with dietary fiber, which helps move food through your digestive tract.

In fact, soybeans are such a good source of food fiber that I feel obligated to add a cautionary note here. One day after I'd read through a bunch of studies about soy's effect on cholesterol levels, I decided to lower my cholesterol level right away. So I had a soy burger for lunch, a half-cup of soybeans and no-fat cheese for an afternoon snack, and another half-cup with tomato sauce at dinner. Delicacy prohibits me from explaining in detail how irritated and upset all that fiber made my digestive tract, but I'm sure you get the picture.

If you choose to use soybeans (or any other dry beans for that matter), take it slow — a little today, a little more tomorrow, and a little bit more the day after that.

## High-quality and low-quality proteins

 Because an animal's body is similar to yours, its proteins contain similar combinations of amino acids. That's why nutritionists call proteins from foods of animal origin — meat, fish, poultry, eggs, and dairy products — *high-quality proteins.* Your body absorbs these proteins more efficiently; they can be used without much waste to synthesize other proteins. The proteins from plants — grains, fruit, vegetables, legumes (beans), nuts, and seeds — often have limited amounts of some amino acids, which means their nutritional content is not as high as animal proteins.

The basic standard against which you measure the value of proteins in food is the egg. Nutrition scientists have arbitrarily given the egg a *biological value* of 100 percent, meaning that, gram for gram, it's the food with the best supply of complete proteins. Other foods that have proportionately more protein may not be as valuable as the egg because they lack sufficient amounts of one or more essential amino acids.

 For example, eggs are 11 percent protein, and dry beans are 22 percent protein. However, the proteins in beans don't provide sufficient amounts of *all* the essential amino acids, so the beans are not as nutritionally complete as proteins from animal foods. The prime exception is the soybean, a legume that's packed with abundant amounts of all the amino acids essential for adults. Soybeans are an excellent source of proteins for vegetarians, especially *vegans,* which are vegetarians who avoid all products of animal origin, including milk and eggs.

The term used to describe the value of the proteins in any one food is *amino acid score*. Because the egg contains all the essential amino acids, it scores 100. Table 3-1 shows the protein quality of representative foods relative to the egg.

| Table 3-1 | Scoring the Amino Acids in Food | |
|---|---|---|
| **Food** | **Protein Content (Grams)** | **Amino Acid Score (Compared to the Egg)** |
| Egg | 33 | 100 |
| Fish | 61 | 100 |
| Beef | 29 | 100 |
| Milk (cow's whole) | 23 | 100 |
| Soybeans | 29 | 100 |
| Dry beans | 22 | 75 |
| Rice | 7 | 62–66 |
| Corn | 7 | 47 |
| Wheat | 13 | 50 |
| Wheat (white flour) | 12 | 36 |

*Source:* Nutritive Value of Foods *(Washington, D.C.: U.S. Department of Agriculture, 1991); George M. Briggs and Doris Howes Calloway,* Nutrition and Physical Fitness, *11th ed. (New York: Holt, Rinehart and Winston, 1984)*

## Complete proteins and incomplete proteins

Another way to describe the quality of proteins is to say that they're either complete or incomplete. A *complete protein* is one that contains ample amounts of all essential amino acids; an *incomplete protein* does not. A protein low in one specific amino acid is called a *limiting protein* because it can build only as much tissue as the smallest amount of the necessary amino acid. You can improve the protein quality in a food containing incomplete/limiting proteins by eating it along with one that contains sufficient amounts of the limited amino acids. Matching foods to create complete proteins is called *complementarity*.

## Homocysteine and your heart

Homocysteine is an *intermediate,* a chemical released when you metabolize (digest) protein. Unlike other amino acids, which are vital to your health, homocysteine can be hazardous to your heart, raising your risk of heart disease by attacking cells in the lining of your arteries by making them reproduce more quickly (the extra cells may block your coronary arteries) or by causing your blood to clot (ditto).

Years and years ago, before cholesterol moved to center stage, some smart heart researchers labeled homocysteine the major nutritional culprit in heart disease. Today, they've been vindicated. The American Heart Association cites high homocysteine levels as an independent probable (but not major) risk factor for heart disease, perhaps explaining why some people with low cholesterol have heart attacks.

But wait! The good news is that information from several studies, including the Harvard/Brigham and Women's Hospital Nurses' Health Study in Boston, suggest that a diet rich in the B vitamin folate lowers blood levels of homocysteine. Most fruits and vegetables have plentiful amounts of folate. Stocking up on them may protect your heart.

# The lowdown on gelatin and your fingernails

Everyone knows that gelatin is protein that strengthens fingernails. Too bad everyone's wrong. Gelatin is produced by treating animal bones with acid, a process that destroys the essential amino acid tryptophan. Surprise: Bananas are high in tryptophan. Slicing bananas onto your gelatin increases the quality of the protein. Adding milk makes it even better, but that still may not heal your splitting nails. The fastest way to a cure is a visit to the dermatologist, who can tell you whether the problem is an allergy to nail polish, too much time spent washing dishes, a medical problem such as a fungal infection, or just plain peeling nails. Then the dermatologist may prescribe a different nail polish (or none at all), protective gloves, a *fungicide* (a drug that wipes out fungi), or a lotion product that strengthens the natural glue that holds the layers of your nails together.

For example, rice is low in the essential amino acid lysine, and beans are low in the essential amino acid methionine. By eating rice with beans, you improve (or complete) the proteins in both. Another example is pasta and cheese. Pasta is low in the essential amino acids lysine and isoleucine; milk products have abundant amounts of these two amino acids. Shaking Parmesan cheese onto pasta creates a higher-quality protein dish. In each case, the foods have complementary amino acids. Other examples of complementary protein dishes are peanut butter with bread, and milk with cereal. Many such combinations are a natural and customary part of the diet in parts of the world where animal proteins are scarce or very expensive. Here are some categories of foods with incomplete proteins:

✔ **Grain foods:** Barley, bread, bulgur wheat, cornmeal, kasha, and pancakes

✔ **Legumes:** Black beans, black-eyed peas, fava beans, kidney beans, lima beans, lentils, peanut butter, peanuts, peas, split peas, and white beans

✔ **Nuts and seeds:** Almonds, Brazil nuts, cashews, pecans, walnuts, pumpkin seeds, sesame seeds (tahini), and sunflower seeds

In order for the foods to complement each other, you must eat them together. In other words, rice and beans at one meal, not rice for lunch and beans for dinner. Table 3-2 shows how to combine foods to improve the quality of their proteins.

| Table 3-2 | How to Combine Foods to Complement Proteins | |
|---|---|---|
| *This Food* | *Complements This Food* | *Examples* |
| Whole grains | Legumes (beans) | Rice and beans |
| Dairy products | Whole grains | Cheese sandwich, pasta with cheese, pancakes (wheat and milk/egg batter) |
| Legumes (beans) | Nuts and/or seeds | Chili soup (beans) with caraway seeds |
| Dairy products | Legumes (beans) | Chili beans with cheese |
| Dairy products | Nuts and seeds | Yogurt with chopped nut garnish |

# Deciding How Much Protein You Need

The National Academy of Sciences Food and Nutrition Board, which sets the requirements for vitamins and minerals, also sets goals for daily protein consumption. As with other nutrients, the board has different recommendations for different groups of people: young or older, men or women.

## Calculating the correct amount

As a general rule, the National Academy of Sciences says healthy people need to get 10 percent to 35 percent of their daily calories from protein. More specifically, the Academy has set a Dietary Reference Intake (DRI) of 45 grams of protein per day for a healthy woman and 52 grams per day for a healthy man.

These amounts are easily obtained from two to three 3-ounce servings of lean meat, fish, or poultry (21 grams each). Vegetarians can get their protein from two eggs (12 to 16 grams), two slices of prepacked fat-free cheese (10 grams), four slices of bread (3 grams each), and 1 cup of yogurt (10 grams).

As you grow older, you synthesize new proteins less efficiently, so your muscle mass (protein tissue) diminishes while your fat content stays the same or rises. This change is why some folks erroneously believe that muscle "turns to fat" in old age. Of course, you still use protein to build new tissue, including hair, skin, and nails, which continue to grow until you cross over into The Great Beyond. By the way, the idea that nails continue to grow after death — a staple of shock movies and horror comics — arises from the fact that after death, tissue around the nails shrinks, making a corpse's nails simply look longer. Who else would let you in on these secrets?

## Dodging protein deficiency

The first sign of protein deficiency is likely to be weak muscles — the body tissue most reliant on protein. For example, children who do not get enough protein have shrunken, weak muscles. They may also have thin hair, their skin may be covered with sores, and blood tests may show that the level of albumin in their blood is below normal. *Albumin* is a protein that helps maintain the body's fluid balance, keeping a proper amount of liquid in and around body cells.

A protein deficiency may also show up in your blood. Red blood cells live for only 120 days. Protein is needed to produce new ones. People who do not get enough protein may become *anemic,* having fewer red blood cells than they need. Protein deficiency may also show up as fluid retention (the big belly on a starving child), hair loss, and muscle wasting caused by the body's attempt to protect itself by digesting the proteins in its own muscle tissue. That's why victims of starvation are, literally, skin and bones.

Given the high protein content of a normal American diet (which generally provides far more protein than you actually require), protein deficiency is rare in the United States except as a consequence of eating disorders such as *anorexia nervosa* (refusal to eat) and *bulimia* (regurgitation after meals).

## Boosting your protein intake: Special considerations

Anyone who's building new tissue quickly needs extra protein. For example, the DRI for protein for women who are pregnant or nursing is 71 grams per day. Injuries also raise your protein requirements. An injured body releases above-normal amounts of protein-destroying hormones from the pituitary and adrenal glands. You need extra protein to protect existing tissues, and after severe blood loss, you need extra protein to make new hemoglobin for red blood cells. Cuts, burns, or surgical procedures mean that you need extra protein to make new skin and muscle cells. Fractures mean extra protein is needed to make new bone. The need for protein is so important when you've been badly injured that if you can't take protein by mouth, you'll be given an intravenous solution of amino acids with glucose (sugar) or emulsified fat.

Do athletes need more proteins than the rest of us? Recent research suggests that the answer may be yes, but athletes easily meet their requirements by increasing the amount of food in their normal diet.

## Avoiding protein overload

Yes, you can get too much protein. Several medical conditions make it difficult for people to digest and process proteins properly. As a result, waste products build up in different parts of the body.

People with liver disease or kidney disease either don't process protein efficiently into urea or don't excrete it efficiently through urine. The result may be uric acid kidney stones or *uremic poisoning* (an excess amount of uric acid in the blood). The pain associated with *gout* (a form of arthritis that affects nine men for every one woman) is caused by uric acid crystals collecting in the spaces around joints. Doctors may recommend a low-protein diet as part of the treatment in these situations.

# Chapter 4

# The Lowdown on Fat and Cholesterol

. . . . . . . . . . . . . . . . . . . . . . . . . . . . . . . . . . .

*In This Chapter*

▶ Assessing the value of fat

▶ Discovering the different kinds of fat in food

▶ Explaining why you need some cholesterol

▶ Balancing the fat (and cholesterol) in your diet

. . . . . . . . . . . . . . . . . . . . . . . . . . . . . . . . . . .

The chemical family name for fats and related compounds such as cholesterol is *lipids* (from *lipos,* the Greek word for fat). Liquid fats are called *oils;* solid fats are called, well, *fat.* With the exception of *cholesterol* (a fatty substance that has no calories and provides no energy), fats are high-energy nutrients. Gram for gram, fats have more than twice as much energy potential (calories) as protein and carbohydrates (affectionately referred to as *carbs*): 9 calories per fat gram versus 4 calories per gram for proteins and carbs.

In this chapter, I cut the fat away from the subject of fats and zero in on the essential facts you need to put together a diet with just enough fat (yes, you do need fat) to provide the bounce that every diet requires. And then I deal with that ultimate baddie — cholesterol. Surprise! You need some of that, too. Onward.

# Finding the Facts about Fat Stuff

Fats are sources of energy that add flavor to food — the sizzle on the steak, you can say. However, as anyone who's spent the last 30 years on planet Earth knows, fats may also be hazardous to your health. The trick is separating the good from the bad. Trust me — it can be done. And this section explains how.

## Understanding how your body uses fat

Here's a sentence that you probably never thought you'd read: A healthy body needs fat. Your body uses *dietary fat* (the fat that you get from food) to make tissue and manufacture biochemicals, such as hormones. Some of the body fat made from food fat is *visible*. Even though your skin covers it, you can *see* the fat in the *adipose* (fatty) *tissue* in female breasts, hips, thighs, buttocks, and belly or male abdomen and shoulders.

This visible body fat

- ✔ Provides a source of stored energy
- ✔ Gives shape to your body
- ✔ Cushions your skin (imagine sitting in a chair for a while to read this book without your buttocks to pillow your bones)
- ✔ Acts as an insulation blanket that reduces heat loss

Other body fat is invisible. You can't see this body fat because it's tucked away in and around your internal organs. This hidden fat is

- ✔ Part of every cell membrane (the outer skin that holds each cell together).

- ✔ A component of *myelin,* the fatty material that sheathes nerve cells and makes it possible for them to fire the electrical messages that enable you to think, see, speak, move, and perform the multitude of tasks natural to a living body; brain tissue also is rich in fat.

- ✔ A shock absorber that protects your organs (as much as possible) if you fall or are injured.

- ✔ A constituent of hormones and other biochemicals, such as vitamin D and bile.

## Pulling energy from fat

Although fat has more energy (calories) per gram than proteins and carbohydrates, your body has a more difficult time pulling the energy out of fatty foods. Imagine a chain of long balloons — the kind people twist into shapes that resemble dachshunds, flowers, and other amusing things. When you drop one of these balloons into water, it floats. That's exactly what happens when you swallow fat-rich foods. The fat floats on top of the watery food-and-liquid mixture in your stomach, which limits the effect that *lipases* — fat-busting digestive enzymes in the mix below — can have on it. Because fat is digested more slowly than proteins and carbohydrates, you feel fuller (a condition called *satiety*) longer after eating high-fat food.

When the fat moves down your digestive tract into your small intestine, an intestinal hormone called *cholestokinin* beeps your gallbladder, signaling for the release of bile. *Bile* is an emulsifier, a substance that enables fat to mix with water so that lipases can start breaking the fat into glycerol and fatty acids. These smaller fragments may be stored in special cells (fat

cells) in adipose tissue, or they may be absorbed
into cells in the intestinal wall, where one of the
following happens:

- They're combined with oxygen (or burned) to
  produce heat/energy, water, and the waste
  product carbon dioxide.

- They're used to make lipoproteins that haul
  fats, including cholesterol, through your
  bloodstream.

Glucose, the molecule you get by digesting carbohydrates, is the body's basic source of energy. Burning
glucose is easier and more efficient than burning fat, so
your body always goes for carbohydrates first. But if
you've used up all your available glucose — maybe
you're stranded in a cabin in the Arctic, you haven't
eaten for a week, a blizzard's howling outside, and the
corner deli 500 miles down the road doesn't deliver —
then it's time to start in on your body fat.

The first step is for an enzyme in your fat cells to
break up stored triglycerides (the form of fat in adipose tissue). The enzyme action releases glycerol and
fatty acids, which travel through your blood to body
cells, where they combine with oxygen to produce
heat/energy, plus water — lots of water — and the
waste product carbon dioxide. As anyone who has
used a high-protein/high-fat/low-carb weight-loss diet
such as the Atkins regimen can tell you, in addition to
all that water, burning fat without glucose produces a
second waste product called ketones. In extreme
cases, high concentrations of ketones (a condition
known as *ketosis*) alter the acid/alkaline balance (or
pH) of your blood and may trip you into a coma. Left
untreated, ketosis can lead to death. Medically, this
condition is most common among people with diabetes. For people on a low-carb diet, the more likely sign
of ketosis is stinky urine or breath that smells like
acetone (nail polish remover).

## *Focusing on the fats in food*

Food contains three kinds of fats: triglycerides, phospholipids, and sterols. Here's how they differ:

- ✔ **Triglycerides:** You use these fats to make adipose tissue and burn for energy.

- ✔ **Phospholipids:** Phospholipids are hybrids — part lipid, part phosphate (a molecule made with the mineral phosphorus) — that act as tiny rowboats, ferrying hormones and fat-soluble vitamins A, D, E, and K through your blood and back and forth in the watery fluid that flows across cell membranes. (By the way, the official name for fluid around cells is *extracellular fluid.* See why I just called it watery fluid?)

- ✔ **Sterols (steroid alcohols):** These are fat and alcohol compounds with no calories. Vitamin D is a sterol. So is the sex hormone testosterone. And so is cholesterol, the base on which your body builds hormones and vitamins.

## *Getting the right amount of fat*

Getting the right amount of fat in your diet is a delicate balancing act. Too much, and you increase your risk of obesity, diabetes, heart disease, and some forms of cancer. (The risk of colon cancer seems to be tied more clearly to a diet high in fat from meat rather than fat from dairy products.) Too little fat, and infants don't thrive, children don't grow, and everyone, regardless of age, is unable to absorb and use fat-soluble vitamins that smooth the skin, protect vision, bolster the immune system, and keep reproductive organs functioning.

In the fall of 2002, the National Academies' Institute of Medicine (IOM) recommended that no more than 20 percent to 45 percent of daily calories should come from fat. On a 2,000-calorie daily diet, that's 400 to 900 calories from fats a day. The *Dietary Guidelines for Americans 2005* (see Chapter 7) lowers that to 20 percent to 30 percent of total calories. Translation: 400 to 600 of the calories on a 2,000-calorie/day regimen.

Because your body doesn't need to get saturated fats, cholesterol, or trans fats from food, neither IOM nor the *Dietary Guidelines for Americans 2005* have set levels for these nutrients, except to say, "Keep them as low as possible, please."

This advice about fat intake is primarily for adults. Although many organizations, such as the American Academy of Pediatrics, the American Heart Association, and the National Heart, Lung, and Blood Institute, recommend restricting fat intake for older children, they stress that infants and toddlers require fatty acids for proper physical growth and mental development, and that's why Mother Nature made human breast milk so high in fatty acids. Never limit the fat in your baby's diet without checking first with your pediatrician.

## Essential fatty acids

An *essential fatty acid* is one that your body needs but cannot assemble from other fats. You have to get it whole, from food. Linoleic acid, found in vegetable oils, is an essential fatty acid. Two others — linolenic acid and arachidonic acid — occupy a somewhat ambiguous position. You can't make them from scratch, but you can make them if you have enough linoleic acid on hand, so food scientists can work up a good fight about whether linolenic and arachidonic acids are actually "essential." In practical terms, who cares?

Linoleic acid is so widely available in food, you're unlikely to experience a deficiency of any of the three — linoleic, linolenic, or arachidonic acids — as long as 2 percent of the calories you get each day come from fat.

In 2002, the IOM published the first daily recommendations for two essential fatty acids, alpha-linolenic acid and linolenic acid. The former is an omega-3 fatty acid (more about that later in this chapter) that's found in fish oils, milk, and some veggie oils. The latter is an omega-6 fatty acid (ditto), found in safflower and corn oil. IOM recommends that

✔ Women get 12 grams linolenic acid and 1.1 grams alpha-linolenic acid per day

✔ Men get 17 grams linolenic acid and 1.6 grams alpha-linolenic acid per day

## Finding fat in all kinds of foods

As a general rule:

✔ Fruits and vegetables have only traces of fat, primarily unsaturated fatty acids.

✔ Grains have small amounts of fat, up to 3 percent of their total weight.

✔ Dairy products vary. Cream is a high-fat food. Regular milks and cheeses are moderately high in fat. Skim milk and skim milk products are low-fat foods. Most of the fat in any dairy product is saturated fatty acids.

✔ Meat is moderately high in fat, and most of its fats are saturated fatty acids.

✔ Poultry (chicken and turkey), without the skin, is relatively low in fat.

✔ Fish may be high or low in fat, primarily unsaturated fatty acids that — lucky for the fish — remain liquid even when the fish is swimming in cold water. (Saturated fats harden when cooled.)

✔ Vegetable oils, butter, and lard are high-fat foods. Most of the fatty acids in vegetable oils are unsaturated; most of the fatty acids in lard and butter are saturated.

✔ Processed foods, such as cakes, breads, canned or frozen meat, and vegetable dishes, are generally higher in fat than plain grains, meats, fruits, and vegetables.

Here's a simple guide to finding which foods are high (or low) in fat. Oils are virtually 100 percent fat. Butter and lard are close behind. After that, the fat level drops, from 70 percent for some nuts down to 2 percent for most bread. The rule to take away from these numbers? A diet high in grains and plants always is lower in fat than a diet high in meat and oils.

## Defining fatty acids and their relationship to dietary fat

Fatty acids are the building blocks of fats. Chemically speaking, a *fatty acid* is a chain of carbon atoms with hydrogen atoms attached and a *carbon-oxygen-oxygen-hydrogen group* (the unit that makes it an acid) at one end.

All the fats in food are combinations of fatty acids. Nutritionists characterize fatty acids as saturated, monounsaturated, or polyunsaturated, depending on how many hydrogen atoms are attached to the carbon atoms in the chain. The more hydrogen atoms, the more saturated the fatty acid. Depending

on which fatty acids predominate, a food fat is like-
wise characterized as saturated, monounsaturated, or
polyunsaturated.

✔ A *saturated fat,* such as butter, has mostly saturated fatty acids. Saturated fats are solid at
   room temperature and get harder when chilled.

✔ A *monounsaturated fat,* such as olive oil, has
   mostly monounsaturated fatty acids.
   Monounsaturated fats are liquid at room temperature; they get thicker when chilled.

✔ A *polyunsaturated fat,* such as corn oil, has
   mostly polyunsaturated fatty acids.
   Polyunsaturated fats are liquid at room temperature; they stay liquid when chilled.

So why is margarine, which is made from unsaturated fats such as corn and soybean oil, a
solid? Because it's been artificially saturated by
food chemists who add hydrogen atoms to
some of its unsaturated fatty acids. This process, known as *hydrogenation,* turns an oil, such
as corn oil, into a solid fat that can be used in
products such as margarines without leaking
out all over the table. A fatty acid with extra
hydrogen atoms is called a *hydrogenated fatty
acid.* Another name for hydrogenated fatty acid
is trans fatty acid. *Trans fatty acids* are not
healthy for your heart. Because of those darned
extra hydrogen atoms, they are, well, more saturated, and they act like — what else? — saturated fats, clogging arteries and raising the
levels of cholesterol in your blood. To make it
easier for you to control your trans fat intake,
the Food and Drug Administration now requires
a new line on the Nutritional Facts label that
tells you exactly how many grams of trans fats
are in any product you buy.

# A nutritional fish story

The good news from a 2002 Harvard survey of more than 43,000 male health professionals shows that the ones who eat 3 to 5 ounces of fish just once a month have a 40 percent lower risk of *ischemic stroke,* a stroke caused by a blood clot in a cranial artery. The Harvard study did not include women, but a report on women and stroke published in the *Journal of the American Medical Association* in 2000 says that women who eat about 4 ounces of fish — think one small can of tuna — two to four times a week appear to cut their risk of stroke by a similar 40 percent.

These benefits are, in large part, because of the presence of *omega-3 fatty acids,* which are unsaturated fatty acids found most commonly in fatty fish such as salmon and sardines. The primary omega-3 is *alpha*-linolenic acid, which your body converts to hormonelike substances called eicosanoids. The *eicosanoids* — eicosapentaenoic acid (EPA) and docosahexaenoic acid (DHA) — reduce inflammation, perhaps by inhibiting an enzyme called COX-2, which is linked to inflammatory diseases such as rheumatoid arthritis (RA). The Arthritis Foundation says omega-3s relieve RA joint inflammation, swelling, and pain.

Omega-3s also are heart-friendly. The fats make the tiny blood particles called platelets less sticky, reducing the possibility that they'll clump together to form blood clots that might obstruct a blood vessel and trigger a heart attack. Omega-3s also knock down levels of bad cholesterol so effectively that the American Heart Association recommends eating fish at least twice a week. Besides, fish also is a good source of *taurine,* an amino acid the journal *Circulation* notes helps maintain the elasticity of blood vessels, which means that the vessels may dilate to permit blood or — horrors! — a blot clot to flow through.

Did I mention that omega-3s are bone builders? Fish oils enable your body to create *calciferol,* a naturally occurring form of vitamin D, the nutrient that enables your body to absorb bone-building calcium — which may be why omega-3s appear to help hold minerals in bone — and increase the formation of new bone.

A pretty kettle of fish, indeed.

You can find respectable amounts of omega-3s in anchovies, haddock, herring, mackerel, salmon, sardines, scallops, tuna (albacore), broccoli, kale, spinach, canola oil, walnut oil, and flaxseed oil.

Here's the other side of the coin: Earlier research suggests that frequent servings of fish may increase the risk of a stroke caused by bleeding in the brain. This situation is common among Native Alaskans who eat plenty of fish and have a higher than normal incidence of hemorrhagic, or bleeding, strokes. The Harvard study found no significant link between fish consumption and bleeding strokes, but researchers say more studies are needed to nail down the relationship — or lack thereof.

Plus, not all omegas are equally beneficial. Omega-6 fatty acids — polyunsaturated fats found in beef, pork, and several vegetable oils, including corn, sunflower, cottonseed, soybean, peanut, and sesame oils — are chemical cousins of omega-3s, but the omega-6s lack the benefits of the omega-3s.

Despite all the benefits fish bring to a healthful diet, my technical editor, University of Maine Food Science Professor Alfred Bushway, wants me to remind you that some fish, particularly those caught in the wild (rather than raised on a fish farm), may be contaminated with metals such as mercury, which has made its way into the water as industrial pollution and may be hazardous for women who are or may be pregnant. Check the food bulletins in your local newspaper or check the FDA's hotline (listed on its Web site, which you can find in Chapter 27) for the most up-to-date data.

Now it's really a pretty kettle of fish!

In the meantime, as I explain in *Controlling Cholesterol For Dummies* (a whole doggone book — published by Wiley — on how to whip your cholesterol profile into shape), the same smart food chemists who invented hydrogenation have now come up with trans fat–free margarines and spreads, including some that are made with plant sterols and stanols.

Plant *sterols* are natural compounds found in oils in grains, fruits, and vegetables, including soybeans, while *stanols* are compounds created by adding hydrogen atoms to sterols from wood pulp and other plant sources. Sterols and stanols work like little sponges, sopping up cholesterol in your intestines before it can make its way into your bloodstream. As a result, your total cholesterol levels and your levels of low-density lipoproteins (otherwise known as LDLs or "bad cholesterol") go down. In some studies, one to two 1-tablespoon servings a day of sterols and stanols can lower levels of bad cholesterol by 10 percent to 17 percent, with results showing up in as little as two weeks. Wow!

Table 4-1 shows the kinds of fatty acids found in some common dietary fats and oils. Fats are characterized according to their predominant fatty acids. For example, as you can plainly see in the table, nearly 25 percent of the fatty acids in corn oil are monounsaturated fatty acids. Nevertheless, because corn oil has more poly-unsaturated fatty acid, corn oil is considered a polyunsaturated fatty acid.

| Table 4-1 | What Fatty Acids Are in That Fat or Oil? | | | |
|---|---|---|---|---|
| Fat or Oil | Saturated Fatty Acid (%) | Monounsaturated Fatty Acid (%) | Polyunsaturated Fatty Acid (%) | Kind of Fat or Oil |
| Canola oil | 7 | 53 | 22 | Monounsaturated |
| Corn oil | 13 | 24 | 59 | Polyunsaturated |
| Olive oil | 14 | 74 | 9 | Monounsaturated |
| Palm oil | 52 | 38 | 10 | Saturated |
| Peanut oil | 17 | 46 | 32 | Monounsaturated |
| Safflower oil | 9 | 12 | 74 | Polyunsaturated |
| Soybean oil | 15 | 23 | 51 | Polyunsaturated |
| Soybean-cottonseed oil | 18 | 29 | 48 | Polyunsaturated |
| Butter | 62 | 30 | 5 | Saturated |
| Lard | 39 | 45 | 11 | Saturated* |

* Because more than one-third of its fats are saturated, nutritionists label lard a saturated fat.

Source: Nutritive Value of Foods (Washington, D.C.: U.S. Department of Agriculture); Food and Life (New York: American Council on Science and Health)

# Considering Cholesterol and You

I mention earlier in this chapter that your body actually *needs* fat, and here's another sentence that may blow your (nutritional) mind: Every healthy body *needs* cholesterol. Look carefully and you find cholesterol in and around your cells, in your fatty tissue, in your organs, and in your glands. What's it doing there? Plenty of useful things. For example, cholesterol

- Protects the integrity of cell membranes

- Helps enable nerve cells to send messages back and forth

- Is a building block for vitamin D (a sterol), made when sunlight hits the fat just under your skin

- Enables your gallbladder to make *bile acids,* digestive chemicals that, in turn, enable you to absorb fats and fat-soluble nutrients such as vitamin A, vitamin D, vitamin E, and vitamin K

- Is a base on which you build steroid hormones such as estrogen and testosterone

## Cholesterol and heart disease

Doctors measure your cholesterol level by taking a sample of blood and counting the milligrams of cholesterol in 1 deciliter (¹⁄₁₀ liter) of blood. When you get your annual report from the doctor, your total cholesterol level looks something like this: 225 mg/dl. Translation: You have 225 milligrams of cholesterol in every tenth of a liter of blood. Why does this matter? Because cholesterol makes its way into blood vessels, sticks to the walls, and forms deposits that eventually block the flow of blood. The more cholesterol you have floating in your blood, the more cholesterol is likely to cross into your arteries, where it may increase your risk of heart attack or stroke.

 As a general rule, the National Cholesterol Education Program (NCEP) says that for adults, a cholesterol level higher than 250 mg/dl is a high risk factor for heart disease; between 200 mg/dl and 250 mg/dl is considered a moderate risk factor; below 200 mg/dl is considered a low risk factor.

 Cholesterol levels alone are not the entire story. Many people with high cholesterol levels live to a ripe old age, but others with low total cholesterol levels develop heart disease. Worse yet, recent research indicates that low cholesterol levels may increase the risk of stroke. In other words, cholesterol is only one of several risk factors for heart disease. Here are some more:

✔ An unfavorable ratio of lipoproteins (see the following section)

✔ Smoking

✔ Obesity

✔ Age (being older is riskier)

✔ Sex (being male is riskier)

✔ A family history of heart disease

To estimate your own risk of heart disease/heart attack, check out the NCEP heart attack risk calculator at http://hin.nhlbi.nih.gov/atpiii/calculator.asp.

# Cholesterol season

Even if you allow yourself to indulge in (a few) high-cholesterol ice cream cones and burgers every day of the year, your cholesterol level may still be naturally lower in the summer than in winter.

The basis for this intriguing culinary conclusion is the 2004 University of Massachusetts SEASONS (Seasonal Variation in Blood Lipids) Study of 517 healthy men and women ages 20 to 70. The volunteers started out with an average cholesterol level of 213 mg/dl (women) to 222 mg/dl (men). A series of five blood tests during the one-year study showed an average drop of 4 points in the summer for men and 5.4 points for women. People with high cholesterol (above 240 mg/dl) did better, dropping as much as 18 points in the summer.

U. Mass. cardiologists say one explanation for the summer downswing may be the normal increase in human blood volume in hot weather. Cholesterol levels reflect the total amount of cholesterol in your bloodstream. With more blood in the stream, the amount of cholesterol per deciliter declines, producing a lower total cholesterol reading. Another possibility: People tend to eat less and be more active in summer. They lose weight, and weight loss equals lower cholesterol.

The first bit of wisdom from this study: Being physically active reduces your cholesterol level. The second: Environment matters. In other words, if you're planning to start a new cholesterol-buster diet, you may do better to start in the winter, when your efforts may lower your total cholesterol as much as 12 points over a reasonable period of time, say, six months. Then when your doctor runs a follow-up test the following summer, you'll get the added benefit of the seasonal slip to make you feel really, really good about how well you're doing. And there's this: For more on controlling your cholesterol, zip out and get yourself a copy of (what else?) my other book, *Controlling Cholesterol For Dummies* (Wiley).

## *Living with lipoproteins*

 A *lipoprotein* is a fat (*lipo* = fat) and protein particle that carries cholesterol through your blood. Your body makes four types of lipoproteins: chylomicrons, very low-density lipoproteins (VLDLs), low-density lipoproteins (LDLs), and high-density lipoproteins (HDLs). As a general rule, LDLs take cholesterol into blood vessels; HDLs carry it out of the body.

A lipoprotein is born as a *chylomicron,* made in your intestinal cells from protein and triglycerides (fats). After 12 hours of traveling through your blood and around your body, a chylomicron has lost virtually all its fats. By the time the chylomicron makes its way to your liver, the only thing left is protein.

The liver, a veritable fat and cholesterol factory, collects fatty acid fragments from your blood and uses them to make cholesterol and new fatty acids. Time out! How much cholesterol you get from food may affect your liver's daily output: Eat more cholesterol, and your liver may make less. If you eat less cholesterol, your liver may make more. And so it goes.

After your liver has made cholesterol and fatty acids, it packages them with protein as very low-density lipoproteins (VLDLs), which have more protein and are denser than their precursors, the chylomicrons. As VLDLs travel through your bloodstream, they lose triglycerides, pick up cholesterol, and turn into low-density lipoproteins (LDLs). LDLs supply cholesterol to your body cells, which use it to make new cell membranes and manufacture sterol compounds such as hormones. That's the good news.

The bad news is that both VLDLs and LDLs are soft and squishy enough to pass through blood vessel walls. The larger and squishier they are, the more likely they are to slide into your arteries, which means that VLDLs are more hazardous to your health than plain old LDLs. These fluffy, fatty lipoproteins carry cholesterol into blood vessels, where it can cling to the inside wall, forming deposits, or *plaques*. These plaques may eventually block an artery, prevent blood from flowing through, and trigger a heart attack or stroke. Whew! Got all that?

VLDLs and LDLs are sometimes called "bad cholesterol," but this characterization is a misnomer. They aren't cholesterol; they're just the rafts on which cholesterol sails into your arteries. Traveling through the body, LDLs continue to lose cholesterol. In the end, they lose so much fat that they become mostly protein — turning them into high-density lipoproteins, the particles sometimes called "good cholesterol." Once again, this label is inaccurate. HDLs aren't cholesterol: They're simply protein and fat particles too dense and compact to pass through blood vessel walls, so they carry cholesterol out of the body rather than into arteries.

That's why a high level of HDLs may reduce your risk of heart attack regardless of your total cholesterol levels. Conversely, a high level of LDLs may raise your risk of heart attack, even if your overall cholesterol level is low. Hey, on second thought, maybe that does qualify them as "good" and "bad" cholesterol.

At one point, back in the dawn of the Cholesterol Age, like, say, five years ago, the "safe" upper limit for LDLs was assumed to be around 160 mg/dl. Now, the National Heart, Lung, and Blood Institute, American College of Cardiology, and the American Heart Association have all put their stamps of approval on the National Cholesterol

Education Program's (NCEP) recommendations for new, lower levels of LDLs based on the presence of the risk factors I list under "Cholesterol and heart disease." You know — diabetes, high blood pressure, obesity . . . those risk factors.

For healthy people with two or more risk factors, the new goal is to push LDLs below 130 mg/dl. For high-risk patients with heart disease or blood vessel problems and more than two risk factors, it's LDLs below 100 mg/dl. For very high-risk patients who are hospitalized with heart disease or have heart disease plus several risk factors, LDLs should be under 70 mg/dl. If necessary, the NCEP suggests using cholesterol-busting statin drugs such as atorvastatin (Lipitor).

## *Diet and cholesterol*

Most of the cholesterol that you need is made right in your own liver, which churns out about 1 gram (1,000 milligrams) a day from the raw materials in the proteins, fats, and carbohydrates that you consume. But you also get cholesterol from food of animal origin: meat, poultry, fish, eggs, and dairy products. Although some plant foods, such as coconuts and cocoa beans, are high in saturated fats, no plants actually have cholesterol. Table 4-2 lists the amount of cholesterol in normal servings of some representative foods.

Because plants don't contain cholesterol, no plant foods are on this list. No grains. No fruits. No veggies. No nuts and seeds. Of course, you can juice plant food up with cholesterol if you really try: Butter in the bread dough, cheese on the macaroni, cream sauce on the peas and onions, whipped cream on poached peaches, and so on.

| Table 4-2 | How Much Cholesterol Is on That Plate? | |
|---|---|---|
| **Food** | **Serving Size** | **Cholesterol (mg)** |
| **Meat** | | |
| Beef (stewed) lean and fat | 3 ounces | 87 |
| Beef (stewed) lean | 2.2 ounces | 66 |
| Beef (ground) lean | 3 ounces | 74 |
| Beef (ground) regular | 3 ounces | 76 |
| Beef steak (sirloin) | 3 ounces | 77 |
| Bacon | 3 strips | 16 |
| Pork chop, lean | 2.5 ounces | 71 |
| **Poultry** | | |
| Chicken (roast) breast | 3 ounces | 73 |
| Chicken (roast) leg | 3 ounces | 78 |
| Turkey (roast) breast | 3 ounces | 59 |
| **Fish** | | |
| Clams | 3 ounces | 43 |
| Flounder | 3 ounces | 59 |
| Oysters (raw) | 1 cup | 120 |
| Salmon (canned) | 3 ounces | 34 |
| Salmon (baked) | 3 ounces | 60 |
| Tuna (water canned) | 3 ounces | 48 |
| Tuna (oil canned) | 3 ounces | 55 |

| Food | Serving Size | Cholesterol (mg) |
|---|---|---|
| **Cheese** | | |
| American | 1 ounce | 27 |
| Cheddar | 1 ounce | 30 |
| Cream | 1 ounce | 31 |
| Mozzarella (whole milk) | 1 ounce | 22 |
| Mozzarella (part skim) | 1 ounce | 15 |
| Swiss | 1 ounce | 26 |
| **Milk** | | |
| Whole | 8 ounces | 33 |
| 2% | 8 ounces | 18 |
| 1% | 8 ounces | 18 |
| Skim | 8 ounces | 10 |
| **Other dairy products** | | |
| Butter | Pat | 11 |
| **Other** | | |
| Eggs, large | 1 | 213 |
| Lard | 1 tbsp. | 12 |

*Source:* Nutritive Value of Foods *(Washington, D.C.: U.S. Department of Agriculture)*

# Chapter 5

# Carbohydrates: A Complex Story

*In This Chapter*
▶ Discovering the different kinds of carbohydrates
▶ Understanding how your body uses carbohydrates
▶ Loading up on carbohydrates before athletic competition
▶ Valuing dietary fiber

*C*arbohydrates — the name means carbon plus water — are sugar compounds that plants make when they're exposed to light. This process of making sugar compounds is called *photosynthesis,* from the Latin words for "light" and "putting together."

In this chapter, I shine a bright light on the different kinds of carbohydrates, illuminating all the nutritional nooks and crannies to explain how each contributes to your vim and vigor — not to mention a yummy daily menu.

# Checking Out Carbohydrates

Carbohydrates come in three varieties: simple carbohydrates, complex carbohydrates, and dietary fiber. All are
composed of units of sugar. What makes one carbohydrate different from another is the number of sugar
units it contains and how the units are linked together.

- **Simple carbohydrates:** These carbohydrates
  have only one or two units of sugar.

  - A carbohydrate with one unit of sugar is called
    a *simple sugar* or a *monosaccharide* (*mono* =
    one; *saccharide* = sugar). Fructose (fruit sugar)
    is a monosaccharide, and so are glucose
    (blood sugar), the sugar produced when you
    digest carbohydrates, and galactose, the sugar
    derived from digesting lactose (milk sugar).

  - A carbohydrate with two units of sugar is
    called a *double sugar* or a *disaccharide* (*di* =
    two). Sucrose (table sugar), which is made of
    one unit of fructose and one unit of glucose,
    is a disaccharide.

- **Complex carbohydrates:** Also known as *polysac-
  charides* (*poly* = many), these carbs have more
  than two units of sugar linked together. Carbs
  with three to ten units of sugar are sometimes
  called *oligosaccharides* (*oligo* = few).

  - Raffinose is a *trisaccharide* (*tri* = three) that's
    found in potatoes, beans, and beets. It has one
    unit each of galactose, glucose, and fructose.

  - Stachyose is a *tetrasaccharide* (*tetra* = four)
    found in the same vegetables mentioned in
    the previous item. It has one fructose unit,
    one glucose unit, and two galactose units.

  - Starch, a complex carbohydrate in potatoes,
    pasta, and rice, is a definite polysaccharide,
    made of many units of glucose.

Because complex carbohydrates are, well, *complex,* with anywhere from three to a zillion units of sugars, your body takes longer to digest them than it takes to digest simple carbohydrates. As a result, digesting complex carbohydrates releases glucose into your bloodstream more slowly and evenly than digesting simple carbs. (For more about digesting carbs, see the section "Carbohydrates and energy: a biochemical love story," later in this chapter.)

✔ **Dietary fiber:** This term is used to distinguish the fiber in food from the natural and synthetic fibers (silk, cotton, wool, nylon) used in fabrics. Dietary fiber is a third kind of carbohydrate.

- Like the complex carbohydrates, dietary fiber (cellulose, hemicellulose, pectin, beta-glucans, gum) is a polysaccharide. Lignin, a different kind of chemical, is also called a dietary fiber.

- Some kinds of dietary fiber also contain units of soluble or insoluble uronic acids, compounds derived from the sugars fructose, glucose, and galactose. For example, pectin — a soluble fiber in apples — contains soluble galacturonic acid.

Dietary fiber is not like other carbohydrates. The bonds that hold its sugar units together cannot be broken by human digestive enzymes. Although the bacteria living naturally in your intestines convert very small amounts of dietary fiber to fatty acids, dietary fiber is not considered a source of energy. (For more about fatty acids, see Chapter 4.)

In the next section, I talk about how your body gets energy from carbohydrates. Because dietary fiber does not provide energy, I'm going to put it aside for

the moment and get back to it in the "Dietary Fiber:
The Non-Nutrient in Carbohydrate Foods" section,
later in this chapter.

## *Carbohydrates and energy:*
## *a biochemical love story*

Your body runs on glucose, the molecules your cells
burn for energy. Proteins, fats, and alcohol (as in beer,
wine, and spirits) also provide energy in the form of calories. And protein does give you glucose, but it takes a
long time, relatively speaking, for your body to get it.

When you eat carbohydrates, your pancreas
secretes insulin, the hormone that enables you
to digest starches and sugars. This release of
insulin is sometimes called an *insulin spike*,
which means the same thing as "insulin secretion" but sounds a whole lot more sinister.

Eating simple carbohydrates such as sucrose (table
sugar) provokes higher insulin secretion than eating
complex carbohydrates such as starch. If you have a
metabolic disorder such as diabetes that keeps you
from producing enough insulin, you must be careful
not to take in more carbs than you can digest.
Unmetabolized sugars circulating through your
blood can make you dizzy and maybe even trip
you into a diabetic coma.

What makes this interesting is that some perfectly
healthful foods, such as carrots, potatoes, and white
bread, have more simple carbs than others, such as
apples, lentils, peanuts, and whole wheat bread. The
Glycemic Index, developed at the University of Toronto
in 1981, gives you a handle on this by ranking foods
according to how quickly they affect blood sugar levels
when compared to glucose (the form of sugar your body
uses as energy), the glycemic indicator *par excellence*.

Most people who don't have a metabolic disorder (such as diabetes) that interferes with the ability to digest carbs can metabolize even very large amounts of carbohydrate foods easily. Their insulin secretion rises to meet the demand and then quickly settles back to normal. In other words, although some popular weight loss programs, such as the South Beach Diet, rely on the Glycemic Index as a weight loss tool, the fact remains that for most people, a carb is a carb is a carb, regardless of how quickly the sugar enters the bloodstream.

For info on why the difference between simple and complex carbs can matter for athletes, check out the section called "Who needs extra carbohydrates?"

## *How glucose becomes energy*

Inside your cells, the glucose is burned to produce heat and *adenosine triphosphate,* a molecule that stores and releases energy as required by the cell. By the way, nutrition scientists, who have as much trouble pronouncing polysyllabic words as you probably do, usually refer to adenosine triphosphate by its initials: ATP. Smart cookies!

The transformation of glucose into energy occurs in one of two ways: with oxygen or without it. Glucose is converted to energy with oxygen in the *mitochondria* — tiny bodies in the jellylike substance inside every cell. This conversion yields energy (ATP, heat) plus water and carbon dioxide — a waste product.

Red blood cells do not have mitochondria, so they change glucose into energy without oxygen. This yields energy (ATP, heat) and lactic acid.

Glucose is also converted to energy in muscle cells. When it comes to producing energy from glucose, muscle cells are, well, double-jointed. They have mitochondria, so they can process glucose with oxygen.

But if the level of oxygen in the muscle cell falls very low, the cells can just go ahead and change glucose into energy without it. This is most likely to happen when you've been exercising so strenuously that you (and your muscles) are, literally, out of breath.

Being able to turn glucose into energy without oxygen is a handy trick, but here's the downside: One byproduct is lactic acid. Why is that a big deal? Too much lactic acid makes your muscles ache.

## How pasta ends up on your hips when too many carbs pass your lips

Your cells budget energy very carefully. They do not store more than they need right now. Any glucose the cell does not need for its daily work is converted to glycogen (animal starch) and tucked away as stored energy in your liver and muscles.

Your body can pack about 400 grams (14 ounces) of glycogen into liver and muscle cells. A gram of carbohydrates — including glucose — has 4 calories. If you add up all the glucose stored in glycogen to the small amount of glucose in your cells and blood, it equals about 1,800 calories of energy.

If your diet provides more carbohydrates than you need to produce this amount of stored calories in the form of glucose and glycogen in your cells, blood, muscles, and liver, the excess will be converted to fat. And that's how your pasta ends up on your hips.

## Other ways your body uses carbohydrates

Providing energy is an important job, but it isn't the only thing carbohydrates do for you. Carbohydrates also protect your muscles. When you need energy, your body looks for glucose from carbohydrates first. If none is available, because you're on a carbohydrate-restricted diet or have a medical condition that prevents you from using the carbohydrate foods you consume, your body begins to pull energy out of fatty tissue and then moves on to burning its own protein tissue (muscles). If this use of proteins for energy continues long enough, you run out of fuel and die.

A diet that provides sufficient amounts of carbohydrates keeps your body from eating its own muscles. That's why a carbohydrate-rich diet is sometimes described as *protein sparing*.

What else do carbohydrates do? They

- Regulate the amount of sugar circulating in your blood so that all your cells get the energy they need
- Provide nutrients for the friendly bacteria in your intestinal tract that help digest food
- Assist in your body's absorption of calcium
- May help lower cholesterol levels and regulate blood pressure (these effects are special benefits of dietary fiber, which I discuss in the "Dietary Fiber: The Non-Nutrient in Carbohydrate Foods" section, later in this chapter)

## Finding the carbohydrates you need

The most important sources of carbohydrates are plant foods — fruits, vegetables, and grains. Milk and milk products contain the carbohydrate lactose (milk sugar), but meat, fish, and poultry have no carbohydrates at all.

In the fall of 2002, the National Academy of Sciences Institute of Medicine (IOM) released a report recommending that 45 percent to 65 percent of your daily

calories come from carbohydrate foods. The Food
Guide Pyramid (see more about that in Chapter 8)
makes it easy for you to build a nutritious carb-based
diet with portion allowances based on how many
calories you consume each day in

- 6 to 11 servings of grain foods (bread, cereals,
  pasta, rice), plus
- 2 to 4 servings of fruit and
- 3 to 5 servings of vegetables

These foods provide simple carbohydrates, complex
carbohydrates, and the natural bonus of dietary fiber.
Table sugar, honey, and sweets — which provide
simple carbohydrates — are recommended only on a
once-in-a-while basis.

One gram of carbohydrates has four calories. To
find the number of calories from the carbohydrates in a serving, multiply the number of
grams of carbohydrates by four. For example,
one whole bagel has about 38 grams of carbohydrates, equal to about 152 calories (38 × 4). (You
have to say "about" because the dietary fiber in
the bagel provides no calories, because the
body can't metabolize it.) *Wait:* That number
does not account for all the calories in the serving. Remember, the foods listed here may also
contain at least some protein and fat, and these
two nutrients add calories.

## Some problems with carbohydrates

Some people have a hard time handling carbohydrates.
For example, people with Type 1 ("insulin dependent")
diabetes do not produce sufficient amounts of insulin,
the hormones needed to carry all the glucose produced
from carbohydrates into body cells. As a result, the
glucose continues to circulate in the blood until it's

excreted through the kidneys. That's why one way to tell whether someone has diabetes is to test the level of sugar in that person's urine.

Other people can't digest carbohydrates because their bodies lack the specific enzymes needed to break the bonds that hold a carbohydrate's sugar units together. For example, many (some say most) Asians, Africans, Middle Easterners, South Americans, and Eastern, Central, or Southern Europeans are deficient in lactase, the enzyme that splits lactose (milk sugar) into glucose and galactose. If they drink milk or eat milk products, they end up with a lot of undigested lactose in their intestinal tracts. This undigested lactose makes the bacteria living there happy as clams — but not the person who owns the intestines: As bacteria feast on the undigested sugar, they excrete waste products that give their host gas and cramps.

 A solution for people who don't make enough lactase is to use a *predigested milk product* such as yogurt or buttermilk or sour cream, all made by adding friendly bacteria that digest the milk (that is, break the lactose apart) without spoiling it. Other solutions include lactose-free cheeses and enzyme-treated milk.

## Who needs extra carbohydrates?

The small amount of glucose in your blood and cells provides the energy you need for your body's daily activities. The 400 grams of glycogen stored in your liver and muscles provides enough energy for ordinary bursts of extra activity.

But what happens when you have to work harder or longer than that? For example, what if you're a long-distance athlete, which means that you use up your available supply of glucose before you finish your competition? (That's why marathoners often run out of gas — a phenomenon called *hitting the wall* — at 20 miles, 6 miles short of the finish line.)

If you were stuck on an ice floe or lost in the woods for a month or so, after your body exhausted its supply of glucose, including the glucose stored in glycogen, it would start pulling energy first out of fat and then out of muscle. But extracting energy from body fat requires large amounts of oxygen — which is likely to be in short supply when your body has run, swum, or cycled 20 miles. So athletes have to find another way to leap the wall. Here it is: They load up on carbohydrates in advance.

 *Carbohydrate-loading* is a dietary regimen designed to increase temporarily the amount of glycogen stored in your muscles in anticipation of an upcoming event. You start about a week before the event, says the University of Maine's Alfred A. Bushway, PhD, exercising to exhaustion so your body pulls as much glycogen as possible out of your muscles. Then, for three days, you eat foods high in fat and protein and low in carbohydrates to keep your glycogen level from rising again.

Three days before the big day, reverse the pattern. Now you want to build and conserve glycogen stores. What you need is a diet that's about 70 percent carbohydrates, providing 6 to 10 grams of carbohydrates for every kilogram (2.2 pounds) of body weight for men and women alike. And not just any carbohydrates, mind you. What you want are the complex carbohydrates in starchy foods like pasta and potatoes, rather than the simple ones more prominent in sugary foods like fruit. And of course, candy.

 This carb-loading diet is not for everyday use, nor will it help people competing in events of short duration. It's strictly for events lasting longer than 90 minutes.

What about while you're running, swimming, or cycling? Will consuming simple sugars during the race give you extra short-term bursts of energy? Yes. Sugar is rapidly converted to glycogen and carried to the muscles. But you don't want *straight sugar* (candy, honey) because it's *hydrophilic* (*hydro* = water; *philic* = loving), which means that it pulls water from body tissues into your intestinal tract. Using straight sugar can increase dehydration and make you nauseated. Thus, getting the sugar you want from sweetened athletic drinks, which provide fluids along with the energy, is best. The label on the athletic drink also tells you the liquid contains salt (sodium chloride). Why? To replace the salt that you lose when perspiring heavily. Turn to Chapter 6 to find out why this is important.

# Dietary Fiber: The Non-Nutrient in Carbohydrate Foods

*Dietary fiber* is a group of complex carbohydrates that are not a source of energy for human beings. Because human digestive enzymes cannot break the bonds that hold fiber's sugar units together, fiber adds no calories to your diet and cannot be converted to glucose.

But just because you can't digest dietary fiber doesn't mean it isn't a valuable part of your diet. The opposite is true. Dietary fiber is valuable *because* you can't digest it!

## The two kinds of dietary fiber

Nutritionists classify dietary fiber as either insoluble fiber or soluble fiber, depending on whether it dissolves in water. (Both kinds of fiber resist human digestive enzymes.)

✔ **Insoluble fiber:** This type of fiber includes cellulose, some hemicelluloses, and lignin found in whole grains and other plants. This kind of dietary fiber is a natural laxative. It absorbs water, helps you feel full after eating, and stimulates your intestinal walls to contract and relax. These natural contractions, called *peristalsis,* move solid materials through your digestive tract.

By moving food quickly through your intestines, insoluble fiber may help relieve or prevent digestive disorders such as constipation or diverticulitis (infection that occurs when food gets stuck in small pouches in the wall of the colon). Insoluble fiber also bulks up stool and makes it softer, reducing your risk of developing hemorrhoids and lessening the discomfort if you already have them.

✔ **Soluble fiber:** This fiber, such as pectins in apples and beta-glucans in oats and barley, seems to lower the amount of cholesterol circulating in your blood (your *cholesterol level*). This tendency may be why a diet rich in fiber appears to offer some protection against heart disease.

Here's a benefit for dieters: Soluble fiber forms gels in the presence of water, which is what happens when apples and oat bran reach your digestive tract. Like insoluble fiber, soluble fiber can make you feel full without adding calories.

## Getting fiber from food

You find fiber in all plant foods — fruits, vegetables, and grains. But you find absolutely no fiber in foods from animals: meat, fish, poultry, milk, milk products, and eggs.

A balanced diet with lots of foods from plants gives you both insoluble and soluble fiber. Most foods that contain fiber have both kinds, although the balance usually tilts toward one or the other. For example, the predominant fiber in an apple is pectin (a soluble fiber), but an apple peel also has some cellulose, hemicellulose, and lignin.

Table 5-1 shows you which foods are particularly good sources of specific kinds of fiber. A diet rich in plant foods (fruits, vegetables, grains) gives you adequate amounts of dietary fiber.

| Table 5-1 | Sources of Different Kinds of Fiber |
|---|---|
| *Fiber* | *Where Found* |
| **Soluble fiber** | |
| Pectin | Fruits (apples, strawberries, citrus fruits) |
| Beta-glucans | Oats, barley |
| Gums | Beans, cereals (oats, rice, barley), seeds, seaweed |
| **Insoluble fiber** | |
| Cellulose | Leaves (cabbage), roots (carrots, beets), bran, whole wheat, beans |
| Hemicellulose | Seed coverings (bran, whole grains) |
| Lignin | Plant stems, leaves, and skin |

## How much fiber do you need?

According to the U.S. Department of Agriculture, the average American woman gets about 12 grams of fiber a day from food; the average American man, 17 grams. Those figures are well below the new IOM (Institute of Medicine) recommendations that I conveniently list here:

- ✔ 25 grams a day for women younger than 50
- ✔ 38 grams a day for men younger than 50
- ✔ 21 grams a day for women older than 50
- ✔ 30 grams a day for men older than 50

The amounts of dietary fiber recommended by IOM are believed to give you the benefits you want without causing fiber-related — um — unpleasantries.

Unpleasantries? Like what? And how will you know if you've got them?

Trust me: If you eat more than enough fiber, your body will tell you right away. All that roughage may irritate your intestinal tract, which will issue an unmistakable protest in the form of intestinal gas or diarrhea. In extreme cases, if you don't drink enough liquids to moisten and soften the fiber you eat so that it easily slides through your digestive tract, the dietary fiber may form a mass that can end up as an intestinal obstruction (for more about water, see Chapter 6).

If you decide to up the amount of fiber in your diet, follow this advice:

- ✔ Do so *very* gradually, a little bit more every day. That way you're less likely to experience intestinal distress.
- ✔ Always check the nutrition label whenever you shop (for more about the wonderfully informative guides, see Chapter 8). When choosing between similar products, just take the one with the higher fiber content per serving.

✔ Get enough liquids. Dietary fiber is like a sponge. It sops up liquid, so increasing your fiber intake may deprive your cells of the water they need to perform their daily work (for more about how your body uses the water you drink, see Chapter 6). That's why the American Academy of Family Physicians (among others) suggests checking to make sure you get plenty fluids when you consume more fiber. How much is enough? Back to Chapter 6.

Table 5-2 shows the amounts of all types of dietary fiber — insoluble plus soluble — in a 100-gram (3.5-ounce) serving of specific foods. By the way, nutritionists like to measure things in terms of 100-gram portions because that makes comparing foods at a glance possible.

To find the amount of dietary fiber in your own serving, you can look at the nutrition label on the side of the package that gives the nutrients per portion.

Finally, the amounts on this chart are averages. Different brands of processed products (breads, some cereals, cooked fruits, and vegetables) may have more (or less) fiber per serving.

| Table 5-2 | Fiber Content in Common Foods |
|---|---|
| *Food* | *Grams of Fiber in a 100-Gram (3.5-Ounce) Serving* |
| **Bread** | |
| Bagel | 2.1 |
| Bran bread | 8.5 |
| Pita bread (white) | 1.6 |

*(continued)*

### Table 5-2 *(continued)*

| Food | Grams of Fiber in a 100-Gram (3.5-Ounce) Serving |
| --- | --- |
| Pita bread (whole wheat) | 7.4 |
| White bread | 1.9 |
| **Cereals** | |
| Bran cereal | 35.3 |
| Bran flakes | 18.8 |
| Cornflakes | 2.0 |
| Oatmeal | 10.6 |
| Wheat flakes | 9.0 |
| **Grains** | |
| Barley, pearled (minus its outer covering), raw | 15.6 |
| Cornmeal, whole grain | 11.0 |
| De-germed | 5.2 |
| Oat bran, raw | 6.6 |
| Rice, raw (brown) | 3.5 |
| Rice, raw (white) | 1.0–2.8 |
| Rice, raw (wild) | 5.2 |
| Wheat bran | 15.0 |
| **Fruits** | |
| Apple, with skin | 2.8 |
| Apricots, dried | 7.8 |
| Figs, dried | 9.3 |
| Kiwi fruit | 3.4 |
| Pear, raw | 2.6 |

| Food | Grams of Fiber in a 100-Gram (3.5-Ounce) Serving |
|------|--------------------------------------------------|
| Prunes, dried | 7.2 |
| Prunes, stewed | 6.6 |
| Raisins | 5.3 |
| **Vegetables** | |
| Baked beans (vegetarian) | 7.7 |
| Chickpeas (canned) | 5.4 |
| Lima beans, cooked | 7.2 |
| Broccoli, raw | 2.8 |
| Brussels sprouts, cooked | 2.6 |
| Cabbage, white, raw | 2.4 |
| Cauliflower, raw | 2.4 |
| Corn, sweet, cooked | 3.7 |
| Peas with edible pods, raw | 2.6 |
| Potatoes, white, baked, w/ skin | 5.5 |
| Sweet potato, cooked | 3.0 |
| Tomatoes, raw | 1.3 |
| **Nuts** | |
| Almonds, oil-roasted | 11.2 |
| Coconut, raw | 9.0 |
| Hazelnuts, oil-roasted | 6.4 |
| Peanuts, dry-roasted | 8.0 |
| Pistachios | 10.8 |

*(continued)*

### Table 5-2 *(continued)*

| Food | Grams of Fiber in a 100-Gram (3.5-Ounce) Serving |
| --- | --- |
| **Other** | |
| Corn chips, toasted | 4.4 |
| Tahini (sesame seed paste) | 9.3 |
| Tofu | 1.2 |

*Source:* Provisional Table on the Dietary Fiber Content of Selected Foods *(Washington, D.C.: U.S. Department of Agriculture, 1988)*

# Chapter 6

# Water Works

. . . . . . . . . . . . . . . . . . . . . . . . . . . . . .

## In This Chapter

▶ Understanding why you need water

▶ Finding out where you get the water you need

▶ Deciding exactly how much water you need

▶ Discovering the nature and functions of electrolytes

. . . . . . . . . . . . . . . . . . . . . . . . . . . . . .

*Y*our body is mostly (50 percent to 70 percent) water. Exactly how much water depends on how old you are and how much muscle and fat you have. Muscle tissue has more water than fat tissue. Because the average male body has proportionately more muscle than the average female body, it also has more water. For the same reason — more muscle — a young body has more water than an older one.

You definitely won't enjoy the experience, but if you have to, you can live without food for weeks at a time, getting subsistence levels of nutrients by digesting your own muscle and fat. But water's different. Without it, you'll die in a matter of days — more quickly in a place warm enough to make you perspire and lose water more quickly.

This chapter clues you in on why water is so important, not to mention how you can manage to keep your body's water level, well, level.

# Investigating the Many Ways Your Body Uses Water

Water is a solvent. It dissolves other substances and carries nutrients and other materials (such as blood cells) around the body, making it possible for every organ to do its job. You need water to

- ✔ **Digest food,** dissolving nutrients so that they can pass through the intestinal cell walls into your bloodstream, and move food along through your intestinal tract

- ✔ **Carry waste products out of your body**

- ✔ **Provide a medium in which biochemical reactions such as metabolism (digesting food, producing energy, and building tissue) occur**

- ✔ **Send electrical messages between cells** so that your muscles can move, your eyes can see, your brain can think, and so on

- ✔ **Regulate body temperature** — cooling your body with moisture (perspiration) that evaporates on your skin

- ✔ **Lubricate your moving parts**

# Maintaining the Right Amount of Water in Your Body

As much as three-quarters of the water in your body is in *intracellular fluid,* the liquid inside body cells. The rest is in *extracellular fluid,* which is all the other body liquids, such as

- ✔ Interstitial fluid (the fluid between cells)
- ✔ Blood plasma (the clear liquid in blood)

> ✔ *Lymph* (a clear, slightly yellow fluid collected
>   from body tissues that flows through your lymph
>   nodes and eventually into your blood vessels)
>
> ✔ Bodily secretions such as sweat, seminal fluid,
>   and vaginal fluids
>
> ✔ Urine

A healthy body has just the right amount of fluid
inside and outside each cell, a situation medical
folk call *fluid balance.* Maintaining your fluid balance is essential to life. If too little water is
inside a cell, it shrivels and dies. If there's too
much water, the cell bursts.

## A balancing act: The role of electrolytes

Your body maintains its fluid balance through the
action of substances called *electrolytes,* which are
mineral compounds that, when dissolved in water,
become electrically charged particles called *ions.*

Many minerals, including calcium, phosphorus, and
magnesium, form compounds that dissolve into
charged particles. But nutritionists generally use the
term *electrolyte* to describe sodium, potassium, and
chlorine. The most familiar electrolyte is the one
found on every dinner table: sodium chloride — plain
old table salt. (In water, its molecules dissolve into
two ions: one sodium ion and one chloride ion.)

Under normal circumstances, the fluid inside your cells
has more potassium than sodium and chloride. The
fluid outside is just the opposite: more sodium and chloride than potassium. The cell wall is a *semipermeable
membrane;* some things pass through, but others don't.
Water molecules and small mineral molecules flow
through freely, unlike larger molecules such as proteins.

The process by which sodium flows out and potassium flows in to keep things on an even keel is called the *sodium pump*. If this process were to cease, sodium ions would build up inside your cells. Sodium attracts water; the more sodium there is inside the cell, the more water flows in. Eventually, the cell would burst and die. The sodium pump, regular as a clock, prevents this imbalance from happening so you can move along, blissfully unaware of those efficient, electric ions.

## Fluoridated water: The real Tooth Fairy

Except for the common cold, dental cavities are the most common human medical problem.

You get cavities from *mutans streptococci,* bacteria that live in dental plaque. The bacteria digest and ferment carbohydrate residue on your teeth (plain table sugar is the worst offender) leaving acid that eats away at the mineral surface of the tooth. This eating away is called *decay*. When the decay gets past the enamel to the softer pulp inside of the tooth, your tooth hurts. And you head for the dentist even though you hate it so much you'd almost rather put up with the pain. But almost doesn't count, so off you go.

Brushing and flossing help prevent cavities by cleaning your teeth so that bacteria have less to feast on. Another way to reduce your susceptibility to cavities is to drink *fluoridated water* — water containing the mineral fluorine.

*Fluoride* — the form of fluorine found in food and water — combines with other minerals in teeth and makes the minerals less soluble (harder to dissolve). You get the most benefit by drinking water containing 1 part fluoride to every 1 million parts water (1 ppm) from the day you're born until the day you get your last permanent tooth, usually around age 11 to 13.

Some drinking water, notably in the American Southwest, is fluoridated naturally when it flows through rocks containing fluorine. Sometimes so much fluoride is in this water that it causes a brownish spotting (or mottling) that occurs while teeth are developing and accumulating minerals. This effect doesn't occur with drinking water artificially supplemented with fluoride at the approved standard of one part fluoride to every million parts of water.

Because fluorides concentrate in bones, some people believe that drinking fluoridated water raises the risk of bone cancers, but no evidence to support this claim has ever been found in human beings. However, in 1990, a U.S. Public Health Service's National Toxicology Program (NTP) study of the long-term effects of high fluoride consumption on laboratory rats and mice added fuel to the fire: Four of the 1,044 laboratory rats and mice fed high doses of fluoride for two years developed *osteosarcoma,* a form of bone cancer.

The study sent an immediate *frisson* (shiver of fear) through the health community, but within a year, federal officials reviewing the study issued an opinion endorsing the safety and effectiveness of fluoridated water.

Here's why: First, the number of cancers among the laboratory animals was low enough to have occurred simply by chance. Second, the cancers occurred only in male rats; no cases were reported in female rats or mice of either sex. Finally, the amount of fluorides the animals ingested was 50 to 100 times higher than what you get in drinking water. To get as much fluoride as those rats did, human beings would have to drink more than 380 8-ounce glasses of fluoridated water a day.

Today, more than half the people living in the United States have access to adequately fluoridated public water supplies. The result is a lifelong 50 percent to 70 percent reduction in cavities among the residents of these communities.

# What else do those electrolytes do?

In addition to keeping fluid levels balanced, sodium, potassium, and chloride ions create electrical impulses that enable cells to send messages back and forth between themselves so you can think, see, move, and perform all the bioelectrical functions that you take for granted.

Sodium, potassium, and chloride are also major minerals and essential nutrients. Like other nutrients, they're useful in these bodily processes:

✔ Sodium helps digest proteins and carbohydrates and keeps your blood from becoming too acidic or too alkaline.

✔ Potassium is used in digestion to synthesize proteins and starch and is a major constituent of muscle tissue.

✔ Chloride is a constituent of hydrochloric acid, which breaks down food in your stomach. It's also used by white blood cells to make *hypochlorite,* a natural antiseptic.

## *Dehydrating without enough water and electrolytes*

Drink more water than you need, and your healthy body simply shrugs its shoulders, so to speak, urinates more copiously, and readjusts the water level. It's hard for a healthy person on a normal diet to drink himself to death on water.

But if you don't get enough water, your body lets you know pretty quickly. The first sign is thirst, that unpleasant dryness in your mouth caused by the loss of water from cells in your gums, tongue, and cheeks. The second sign is reduced urination.

Reduced urination is a protective mechanism triggered by *antidiuretic hormone* (ADH), which is secreted by the hypothalamus, a gland at the base of your brain. A diuretic is a substance, such as caffeine, that increases urine production. ADH does just the opposite, helping your body conserve water rather than eliminate it.

If you don't heed these signals, your tissues will begin to dry out. In other words, you're dehydrating, and if you don't — or can't — get water, you won't survive.

# *Getting the Water You Need*

Because you don't store water, you need to take in a new supply every day, enough to replace what you lose when you breathe, perspire, urinate, and defecate. On average, this needed amount adds up to 50 to 100 ounces (6 to 12½ cups) a day. Of this, 28 to 40 ounces is lost in breath and perspiration, 20 to 53 ounces is lost in urine, and 1.6 to 6.6 ounces is lost in feces. Toss in some extra ounces for a safe margin, and you get the current recommendations that women age 19 and up consume about 11 cups of water a day and men age 19 and up, about 15.

But not all that water must come in a cup from the tap. About 15 percent of the water that you need is created when you digest and metabolize food. The end products of digestion and metabolism are carbon dioxide (a waste product that you breathe out of your body) and water composed of hydrogen from food and oxygen from the air that you breathe.

The rest of your daily water comes directly from what you eat and drink. You can get water from, well, plain water. Eight 10-ounce glasses give you approximately enough to replace what your body loses every day, so everyone from athletes to couch potatoes knows that a healthy body needs eight full glasses of water a day.

# Death by dehydration: Not a pretty sight

Every day, you lose an amount of water equal to about 4 percent of your total weight. If you don't take in enough water to replace what you lose naturally by breathing, perspiring, urinating, and defecating, warning signals go off loud and clear.

Early on, when you've lost just a little water, equal to about 1 percent of your body weight, you feel thirsty. If you ignore thirst, it grows more intense.

When water loss rises to about 2 percent of your weight, your appetite fades. Your circulation slows as water seeps out of blood cells and blood plasma. And you experience a sense of emotional discomfort, a perception that things are, well, not right.

By the time your water loss equals 4 percent of your body weight (5 pounds for a 130-pound woman; 7 pounds for a 170-pound man), you're slightly nauseated, your skin is flushed, and you're very, very tired. With less water circulating through your tissues, your hands and feet tingle, your head aches, your temperature rises, you breathe more quickly, and your pulse quickens.

After this, things begin spiraling downhill. When your water loss reaches 10 percent of your body weight, your tongue swells, your kidneys start to fail, and you're so dizzy that you can't stand on one foot with your eyes closed. In fact, you probably can't even try: Your muscles are in spasm.

When you lose enough water to equal 15 percent of your body weight, you're deaf and pretty much unable to see out of eyes that are sunken and covered with stiffened lids. Your skin has shrunk, and your tongue has shriveled.

When you've lost water equal to 20 percent of your body weight, you've had it. You're at the limit of your endurance. Deprived of life-giving liquid, your skin cracks, and your organs grind to a halt. And — sorry about this — so do you. *Ave atque vale,* as the Romans say. Or as the Romans say when in the U.S., Canada, Great Britain, Australia, or any place where English is the mother tongue: "Hail and farewell."

Or at least they thought they knew, but then Dartmouth Medical School kidney specialist Heinz Valtin turned off the tap. Yes, the National Research Council's Food and Nutrition Board says each of us needs about 1 milliliter (ml) of water for each calorie of food we consume. On a 2,000-calorie-a-day diet, that's about 74 fluid ounces, or slightly more than nine 8-ounce glasses a day. Fair enough, Valtin said, but who says that it all has to come from, well, water? His report in the *American Journal of Physiology* (2003) points out that some of the water you require is right there in your food. Fruits and vegetables are full of water. Lettuce, for example, is 90 percent water. Furthermore, you get water from foods that you'd never think of as water sources: hamburger (more than 50 percent), cheese (the softer the cheese, the higher the water content — Swiss cheese is 38 percent water; skim-milk ricotta, 74 percent), a plain, hard bagel (29 percent water), milk powder (2 percent), and even butter and margarine (10 percent). Only oils have no water.

In other words (actually in Valtin's words), a healthy adult in a temperate climate who isn't perspiring heavily can get enough water simply by drinking only when he's

thirsty. Gulp. Or by drinking water when he's also drinking lots of coffee, tea, soft drinks, or alcohol.

 Not all liquids are equally liquefying. The caffeine
in coffee and tea and the alcohol in beer, wine,
and spirits are *diuretics,* chemicals that make you
urinate more copiously. Although caffeinated and
alcoholic beverages provide water, they also
increase its elimination from your body — which
is why you feel thirsty the morning after you've
had a glass or two of wine. And when you feel
thirsty, what do you do? Drink some water.

## Taking in Extra Water and Electrolytes as Needed

In the United States, most people regularly consume
much more sodium than they need. In fact, some
people who are sodium-sensitive may end up with
high blood pressure that can be lowered if they
reduce their sodium intake. (For more about high
blood pressure, check out *High Blood Pressure For
Dummies,* by Alan L. Rubin, MD [Wiley].)

Potassium and chloride are found in so many foods
that here, too, a dietary deficiency is a rarity. In fact,
the only recorded case of chloride deficiency was
among infants given a formula liquid from which the
chloride was inadvertently omitted.

 In 2004, the Adequate Intake (AI) for sodium,
potassium, and chloride were set at one-size-
fits-all averages for a healthy adult age 19 to 50
weighing 154 pounds:

  ✔ **Sodium:** 1,500 milligrams

  ✔ **Potassium:** 4,700 milligrams

  ✔ **Chloride:** 2,300 milligrams

Most Americans get much more as a matter of course, and sometimes you actually need extra water and electrolytes. The next sections tell you when.

## How does water know where to go?

*Osmosis* is the principle that governs how water flows through a semipermeable membrane (one that lets only certain substances pass through) such as the one surrounding a body cell.

Here's the principle: Water flows through a semipermeable membrane from the side where the liquid solution is least dense to the side where it's denser. In other words, the water, acting as if it has a mind of its own, tries to equalize the densities of the liquids on both sides of the membrane.

How does the water know which side is more dense? Now that one's easy: Wherever the sodium content is higher. When more sodium is inside the cell, more water flows in to dilute it. When more sodium is in the fluid outside the cell, water flows out of the cell to dilute the liquid on the outside.

Osmosis explains why drinking seawater doesn't hydrate your body. When you drink seawater, liquid flows out of your cells to dilute the salty solution in your intestinal tract. The more you drink, the more water you lose. When you drink seawater, you're literally drinking yourself into dehydration.

Of course, the same thing happens — though certainly to a lesser degree — when you eat salted pretzels or nuts. The salt in your mouth makes your saliva saltier. This draws liquid out of the cells in your cheeks and tongue, which feel uncomfortably dry. You need . . . a drink of water!

## *You're sick to your stomach*

Repeated vomiting or diarrhea drains your body of
water and electrolytes. Similarly, you also need extra
water to replace the liquid lost in perspiration when
you have a high fever.

# When ginger ale won't cut it

Serious dehydration calls for serious medicine, such as the
World Health Organization's handy-dandy, two-tumbler
electrolyte replacement formula.

Wait! Stop! If you're reading this while lying in bed
exhausted by some variety of *turista,* the traveler's diarrhea
acquired from impure drinking water, do not make the formula without absolutely clean glasses, washed in bottled
water. Better yet, get paper cups.

Now here's what you need:

**Glass No. 1**

8 ounces orange juice

A pinch of salt

½ teaspoon sweetener (honey, corn syrup)

**Glass No. 2**

8 ounces boiled or bottled or distilled water

¼ teaspoon baking soda

Take a sip from one glass, then the other, and continue until
finished. If diarrhea continues, contact your doctor.

When you lose enough water to be dangerously dehydrated, you also lose the electrolytes you need to maintain fluid balance, regulate body temperature, and trigger dozens of biochemical reactions. Plain water doesn't replace those electrolytes. Check with your doctor for a drink that will hydrate your body without upsetting your stomach.

## You're exercising or working hard in a hot environment

When you're warm, your body perspires. The moisture evaporates and cools your skin so that blood circulating up from the center of your body to the surface is cooled. The cooled blood returns to the center of your body, lowering the temperature there (your *core temperature*), too.

If you don't cool down your body, you continue losing water. If you don't replace the lost water, things can get dicey because not only are you losing water, but you're also losing electrolytes. The most common cause of temporary sodium, potassium, and chloride depletion is heavy, uncontrolled perspiration.

Deprived of water and electrolytes, your muscles cramp, you're dizzy and weak, and perspiration, now uncontrolled, no longer cools you. Your core body temperature begins rising, and without relief — air conditioning or a cool shower, plus water, ginger ale, or fruit juice — you may progress from heat cramps to heat exhaustion to heat stroke. And heat stroke is potentially fatal.

But — and it's a big one — drinking *too much* water while exercising can also be hazardous to your health. Flooding your body with liquid dilutes the sodium in your bloodstream and may make your brain and other body tissues swell, a condition known as *hyponaturemia* or "water intoxication." The New Rule from the American College of Sports Medicine is to drink just enough water to maintain your body weight while working out. How much is that? Step on a scale before exercising. Exercise for an hour. Step back on the scale. You need 16 ounces of water to replace every pound lost in your one hour's exercise. Lose 1 pound, drink 16 ounces. Lose ½ pound, drink 8 ounces. That was easy!

# Water is water — or is it?

Chemically speaking, water's an odd duck. It's the only substance on Earth that can exist as a liquid (water) and a solid (ice) — but not a bendable plastic. No, snow is not plastic water. It's a grouping of solids (ice crystals).

Water may be hard or soft, but these terms have nothing to do with how the water feels on your hand. They describe the liquid's mineral content:

- ✔ **Hard water** has lots of minerals, particularly calcium and magnesium. This water rises to the Earth's surface from underground springs, usually picking up calcium carbonate as it moves up through the ground.

- ✔ **Soft water** has fewer minerals. In nature, soft water is surface water, the runoff from rain-swollen streams or rainwater that falls directly into reservoirs. *Water softeners* are products that attract and remove the minerals in water.

What you get at the supermarket is another thing altogether:

✔ **Distilled water** is tap water that has been *distilled,* or boiled until it turns to steam, which is then collected and condensed back into a liquid free of impurities, chemicals, and minerals.

   The name may also be used to describe a liquid produced by *ultrafiltration,* a process that removes everything from the water except water molecules. Distilled water is very important in chemical and pharmaceutical processing. You'll appreciate the fact that it doesn't clog your iron; makes clean, clear ice cubes; and serves as a flavor-free mixer or base for tea and coffee.

✔ **Mineral water** is spring water. It's naturally alkaline, which makes it a natural antacid and a mild *diuretic* (a substance that increases urination). The term **spring water** is used to describe water from springs nearer to the Earth's surface, so it has fewer mineral particles and what some people describe as a "cleaner taste" than mineral water.

✔ **Still water** is spring water that flows up to the surface on its own. **Sparkling water** is pushed to the top by naturally occurring gases in the underground spring. So, you ask, what's the big difference? Sparkling water has bubbles; still water doesn't.

✔ *Springlike* or *spring fresh* are terms designed to make something sound more highfalutin than it really is. These products aren't spring water; they're probably filtered tap water.

## You're on a high-protein diet

You need extra water to eliminate the nitrogen compounds in protein. This is true for infants on high-protein formulas and adults on high-protein
weight-reducing diets. (See Chapter 3 to find out why
too much protein may be so harmful.)

## You're taking certain medications

Because some medications interact with water and
electrolytes, always ask whether you need extra
water and electrolytes whenever your doctor
prescribes

- **Diuretics:** They increase the loss of sodium,
  potassium, and chloride.

- **Neomycin (an antibiotic):** It binds sodium into
  insoluble compounds, making it less available to
  your body.

- **Colchicine (an anti-gout drug):** It lowers your
  absorption of sodium.

## You have high blood pressure

In 1997, when researchers at Johns Hopkins analyzed
the results of more than 30 studies dealing with high
blood pressure, they found that people taking daily
supplements of 2,500 milligrams of potassium were
likely to have blood pressure several points lower
than people not taking the supplements. Ask your
doctor about this one, and remember: Food is also a
good source of potassium. One whole banana has up
to 470 milligrams of potassium; 1 cup of dates, 1,160
milligrams; and 1 cup of raisins, 1,239 milligrams.

# Chapter 7

# What Is a Healthful Diet?

*In This Chapter*

▶ Introducing the *Dietary Guidelines for Americans 2005*

▶ Establishing a healthful lifestyle

▶ Using good judgment when choosing foods

▶ Applying the guidelines realistically

*T*he American Heart Association says to limit your consumption of fats and cholesterol. The American Cancer Society says to eat more fiber. The National Research Council says to watch out for fats, sugar, and salt. The American Diabetes Association says to eat regular meals so your blood sugar stays even. The Food Police say if it tastes good, forget it!

The U.S. Department of Agriculture and Department of Health and Human Services have incorporated virtually all but the "tastes good, forget it" rule into the *Dietary Guidelines for Americans 2005* and even added some advisories of their own.

In this chapter, I give you the information you need to make sure you're following a healthful diet.

# What Are Dietary Guidelines for Americans?

The *Dietary Guidelines for Americans* is a collection of sensible suggestions first published by the U.S. Department of Agriculture (USDA) and Department of Health and Human Services (HHS) in 1980, with five revised editions since then (1985, 1990, 1995, 2000, 2005).

As the first chapter of the 2005 edition explains, the *Guidelines* lays out food and lifestyle choices that promote good health, provide the energy for an active life, and may reduce the risk or severity of chronic illnesses, such as diabetes and heart disease.

# Controlling Your Weight

During the past two decades, as the number of overweight Americans has bounced upward like a rubber ball, the incidence of obesity-related conditions such as Type 2 diabetes, high blood pressure, and heart disease also has risen.

The challenge (as always) is to set, reach, and hold a healthful weight. The new *Dietary Guidelines* lays out some clear, um, guidelines.

## Getting the most nutritious calories

Some foods provide lots of nutrients per calorie; others don't. The former are called *nutrient-dense foods;* the latter aren't.

As you may expect, the *Guidelines* recommends choosing foods from the first group to meet your calorie needs each day, while limiting the amount of

- ✔ Foods high in saturated fat
- ✔ Foods high in trans fats
- ✔ Foods high in cholesterol
- ✔ Foods with added sugar
- ✔ Foods with added salt
- ✔ Alcoholic beverages

In other words, stick to a balanced diet. No surprise there.

## Managing your weight

To reach and keep a healthful weight, follow a few realistic rules:

- ✔ **Evaluate your weight.** The best test of who's actually overweight is the *body mass index* (BMI), a measure of body fat versus body lean mass (in other words, muscle) that can be used to predict health outcomes. To calculate your BMI, go to www.nhlbisupport.com/bmi.

- ✔ **If you need to lose weight, do so gradually.** Forget the "lose 30 pounds in 30 days" jazz. Depending on how much weight you have to lose, your long-term goal needs to be losing about 10 percent of your total weight over a six-month period. Losing ½ to 2 pounds a week is a safe and practical way of doing so.

- ✔ **Encourage healthy weight in children.** One unhappy fact is that overweight kids become overweight adults. Helping children stick to a healthy weight pays large dividends down the road of life.

✔ **Check with your doctor before starting a weight-loss diet.** This advice is most important for women who are pregnant or nursing, for children, and for anyone — young or old — who has a chronic disease and/or is on medication.

## *Being physically active*

When you take in more calories from food than you use up running your body systems (heart, lungs, brain, and so forth) and doing a day's physical work, you end up storing the extra calories as body fat. In other words, you gain weight. The reverse also is true. When you spend more energy in a day than you take in as food, you pull the extra energy you need out of stored fat and you lose weight.

Even being mildly active increases the number of calories you can wolf down without gaining weight. The more strenuous the activity, the more plentiful the calorie allowance.

After you decide to start moving, the *Guidelines* says, do it every day. How much should you do? Per the *Guidelines:*

✔ Most people will benefit from 30 minutes of moderate physical activity — such as a brisk walk — per day.

✔ To manage body weight and/or prevent gradual weight gain, make it 60 minutes of moderate-to-vigorous-intensity activity several days a week.

✔ To keep weight off, try 60 to 90 minutes of daily moderate physical activity.

# Other reasons to exercise

Weight control is a good reason to step up your exercise level, but it isn't the only one. Here are four more:

✔ **Exercise increases muscles.** When you exercise regularly, you end up with more muscle tissue than the average bear. Because muscle tissue weighs more than fat tissue, athletes (even weekend-warrior types) may end up weighing more than they did before they started exercising to lose weight. But a higher muscle-to-fat ratio is healthier and more important in the long run than actual weight in pounds. Exercise that changes your body's ratio of muscle to fat gives you a leg up in the longevity race.

✔ **Exercise reduces the amount of fat stored in your body.** People who are fat around the middle as opposed to the hips (in other words an apple shape versus a pear shape) are at higher risk of weight-related illness. Exercise helps reduce abdominal fat and, thus, lowers your risk of weight-related diseases. Use a tape measure to identify your own body type by comparing your waistline to your hips (around the buttocks). If your waist (abdomen) is bigger, you're an apple. If your hips are bigger, you're a pear.

✔ **Exercise strengthens your bones.** *Osteoporosis* (thinning of the bones that leads to repeated fractures) doesn't happen only to little old ladies. True, on average, a woman's bones thin faster and more dramatically than a man's, but after the mid-30s, everybody — male and female — begins losing bone density. Exercise can slow, halt, or in some cases even reverse the process. In addition, being physically active develops muscles that help support bones. Stronger bones equal less risk of fracture, which, in turn, equals less risk of potentially fatal complications.

*(continued)*

*(continued)*

> ✔ **Exercise increases brainpower.** You know that aerobic
> exercise increases the flow of oxygen to the heart, but
> did you also know that it increases the flow of oxygen to
> the brain?
>
> When a rush job (or a rush of anxiety) keeps you up all
> night, a judicious exercise break can keep you bright
> until dawn. According to Massachusetts Institute of
> Technology nutrition research scientist Judith J.
> Wurtman, PhD, when you're awake and working during
> hours that you'd normally be asleep, your internal body
> rhythms tell your body to cool down, even though your
> brain is racing along. Simply standing up and stretch-
> ing, walking around the room, or doing a couple of sit-
> ups every hour or so speeds up your metabolism,
> warms your muscles, increases your ability to stay
> awake, and, in Dr. Wurtman's words, "prolongs your
> ability to work smart into the night." Eureka!

✔ To reach true physical fitness, your regimen
   should include cardiovascular conditioning,
   stretching exercises for flexibility, and resis-
   tance exercises or calisthenics for muscle
   strength and endurance.

Not everybody can — or should — run right out
and start chopping down trees or throwing
touchdown passes to control his weight. In fact,
if you've gained a lot of weight recently, you've
been overweight for a long time, you haven't exer-
cised in a while, or you have a chronic medical
condition, you need to check with your doctor
before starting any new regimen. (*Caution:*
Check out of any health club that puts you right
on the floor without first checking your vital
signs — heartbeat, respiration, and so forth.)

# Making Smart Food Choices

Okay, so you have your weight goals firmly in mind and three, or four, or even seven times a week, you manage to *Hup! Two, three, four* at home, or in the gym, or on a walk around the block. The next task set forth by the *Guidelines* is to put together a diet that supports your new healthy lifestyle.

## Picking the perfect plants

From the beginning, way back in 1980, the various editions of the *Guidelines* have recommended that you build your diet on a base of plant foods. Why? Because plant foods

- ✔ Add plenty of bulk but few calories to your diet, so you feel full without adding weight

- ✔ Are usually low in fat and have no cholesterol, which means they reduce your risk of heart disease

- ✔ Are high in fiber, which reduces the risk of heart disease; prevents constipation; reduces the risk of developing hemorrhoids (or at least makes existing ones less painful); moves food quickly through your digestive tract, thus reducing the risk of *diverticular disease* (inflammation caused by food getting caught in the folds of your intestines and causing tiny out-pouchings of the weakened gut wall); and may lower your risk of some gastrointestinal cancers

- ✔ Are rich in beneficial substances called phytochemicals, which may reduce your risk of heart disease and some forms of cancer

For all these reasons, the *Guidelines* recommends that a basic 2,000-calorie daily diet include

- 2 cups of fruit

- 2½ cups of vegetables (include dark green, orange, and starchy veggies, plus beans)

- 3 or more 1-ounce servings of whole-grain products

 To protect your bones, the *Guidelines* advises washing down your plants with 3 daily cups of low-fat milk (349 milligrams calcium) or fat-free milk (306 milligrams calcium) or the equivalent amount of milk products such as cheddar cheese, which has 204 milligrams of calcium per ounce.

## Figuring out fats

As you can plainly see in Chapter 4, *dietary fat* (the fat in foods) is an essential nutrient. Infants need these fats to thrive, and the same cholesterol that may increase an adult's risk of heart disease is vital to an embryo's healthy development, triggering the action of genes that tells cells to become specialized body structures — arms, legs, backbone, and so forth.

Grown-ups, however, need to control fat intake so they can control calories and reduce the risk of obesity-related illnesses, such as heart disease, diabetes, and some forms of cancer.

Overall, the *Guidelines* suggests that your adult diet derive no more than 35 percent of its calories from fat and no more than 10 percent of calories from saturated fat and that it deliver 300 milligrams or less of cholesterol a day. To reach these goals

- Most of your fat calories should come from foods such as fish, nuts, and vegetable oils that are rich in polyunsaturated and monounsaturated fats.

✔ Dairy products, such as milk, should be low- or no-fat (skim).

✔ Poultry and meat should be lean. (Yes, trim off that visible fat.)

✔ You should minimize your intake of trans fats. Less is always better.

## Counting on carbs

Carbs are your fastest source of energy, but the trick here is to get your carbs complex (I explain complex versus simple carbs in Chapter 5), which means from plant foods: fruits and vegetables and whole grains. The companion stratagem is to buy and prepare foods with little added sugar.

Together, these two simple steps help control weight, provide vital nutrients, and — as the *Guidelines* slyly notes — "reduce the incidence of dental caries" (cavities). Next!

## Limiting salt, balancing potassium

*Sodium* is a mineral that helps regulate your body's fluid balance, the flow of water into and out of every cell described in Chapter 6. This balance keeps just enough water inside the cell so that it can perform its daily jobs but not so much that the cell — packed to bursting — explodes.

Most people have no problems with sodium. They eat a lot one day, a little less the next, and their bodies adjust. Others, however, don't react so evenly. For them, a high-sodium diet appears to increase the risk of high blood pressure. When you already have high blood pressure, you can tell fairly quickly whether lowering the amount of salt in your diet lowers your blood pressure. But no test is available at this point for telling whether someone who doesn't have high blood pressure will develop it by consuming a diet that's high in sodium.

Because limiting sodium intake to a moderate level won't harm anyone, the *Guidelines* advocates avoiding excessive amounts of salt. Doing so helps reduce blood pressure levels for people who are salt-sensitive.

What's moderate use? According to the *Guidelines,* you should consume less than 2,300 milligrams of sodium per day (that's about 1 teaspoon). The easiest way to reach that goal is to choose and prepare foods with very little added salt. At the same time, it pays to consume potassium-rich foods, such as (what else?) fruits and vegetables, because an adequate supply of potassium helps control blood pressure.

By the way, moderating your salt intake has another, unadvertised benefit. It may lower your weight a bit. Why? Because sodium is *hydrophilic* (*hydro* = water; *philic* = loving). Sodium attracts and holds water. When you eat less salt, you retain less water, you're less bloated, and you feel thinner.

Don't reduce salt intake drastically without first checking with your doctor. ***Remember:*** Sodium is an essential nutrient, and the *Guidelines* advocates moderate use, and not no use at all.

The foods with the highest amounts of naturally occurring sodium are natural cheeses, sea fish, and shellfish. Some foods are low in sodium but pick up plenty of salt when they're processed. For example, 1 cup of cooked fresh green peas has about 2 milligrams of sodium, but 1 cup of canned peas may have 493 milligrams of sodium. To be fair, most canned and processed vegetables are now available in low-sodium versions, too. The difference is notable: A cup of low-sodium canned peas has 8 milligrams of sodium, 485 milligrams less than regular canned peas.

You also get added sodium in the salt on snack foods, such as potato chips and peanuts, not to mention the salt you add yourself from the shaker that's on virtually every American table. Not all the sodium you swallow is sodium chloride. Sodium compounds also are used as preservatives, thickeners, and buffers (chemicals that smooth down acidity).

Table 7-1 lists several different kinds of sodium compounds in food. Table 7-2 lists sodium compounds in over-the-counter drug products.

| Table 7-1 | Sodium Compounds in Food |
|---|---|
| *Sodium Compound* | *Function* |
| Monosodium glutamate (MSG) | Flavor enhancer |
| Sodium benzoate | Keeps food from spoiling |
| Sodium caseinate | Thickens foods and provides protein |
| Sodium chloride (table salt) | Flavoring agent |
| Sodium citrate | Holds carbonation in soft drinks |
| Sodium hydroxide | Makes peeling the skin off tomatoes and fruits before canning easier |
| Sodium nitrate/nitrite | Keeps food (cured meats) from spoiling — and gives these foods their distinctive red color |
| Sodium phosphates | Mineral supplement |
| Sodium saccharin | No-calorie sweetener |

*Source: "The Sodium Content of Your Food,"* Home and Garden Bulletin, *No. 233 (Washington, D.C.: U.S. Department of Agriculture, August 1980); Ruth Winter,* A Consumer's Dictionary of Food Additives *(New York: Crown, 1978)*

| Table 7-2 | Sodium Compounds in Over-the-Counter Drug Products |
|-----------|---------------------------------------------------|
| *Sodium Compound* | *Function* |
| Sodium ascorbate | A form of vitamin C used in nutritional supplements |
| Sodium bicarbonate | Antacid |
| Sodium biphosphate | Laxative |
| Sodium citrate | Antacid |
| Sodium fluoride | Mineral used in nutritional supplements and as a decay preventative in tooth powders |
| Sodium phosphates | Laxative |
| Sodium saccharin | Sweetener |
| Sodium salicylate | Analgesic (similar to aspirin) |

*Source:* Handbook of Nonprescription Drugs, *9th edition (Washington, D.C.: American Pharmaceutical Association, 1990);* Physicians' Desk Reference, *48th edition (Montvale, NJ: Medical Economics Data Production, 1994)*

## *Moderating alcohol consumption*

Telling someone to drink alcohol beverages in moderation sounds like mom-and-apple-pie advice, right? Right. But — and you've heard this song before — what's *moderation,* anyway? Laypersons (you and me, babe) may define *moderate* in terms of the effects that alcohol has on the ability to perform simple tasks, such as speaking and thinking clearly or moving in a straight line. Obviously, if the amount of alcohol you drink makes you slur your words or bump into the furniture, that isn't moderation.

The *Dietary Guidelines* defines moderate drinking as one drink a day for a woman and two drinks a day for a man. Aha, you say, but what's one drink? Good question. Here's the answer, according to the *Guidelines:*

✔ 12 ounces of regular beer (150 calories)

✔ 5 ounces of wine (100 calories)

✔ 1½ ounces of 80-proof (40 percent alcohol) distilled spirits (100 calories)

Some people shouldn't drink at all, not even in moderation, including people who suffer from alcoholism, people who plan to drive a car or take part in other activities that require attention to detail or real physical skill, and people using medication (prescription drugs or over-the-counter products).

# Okay, Now Relax

Life is not a test. You don't lose points for failing to follow the *Dietary Guidelines for Americans 2005* every single day of your life. Nobody's perfect, and the guidelines are meant to be broken — once in a while.

For example, ideally you should hold your daily intake of dietary fat to 20 percent to 35 percent of your total calories. But you can bet that you'll exceed that amount this Saturday when you stroll by the buffet at your best friend's wedding and see Camembert cheese (70 percent of the calories from fat), sirloin steak (56 percent of the calories from fat), salad with Thousand Island dressing (90 percent of the calories from fat), and whipped-cream cake (I can't count that high).

Is this a crisis? Should you stay home? Must you keep your mouth shut tight all night? Are you kidding? Here's the real rule: Let the good times roll every once in a while. After the party's over, compensate: For the rest of the week, go back to your exercise regimen and back to your healthful menu emphasizing lots of the nutritious, delicious, low- or no-fat foods that should make up most of your regular diet.

In the end, you're likely to have averaged out to a desirable amount with no fuss and no muss and be right in line with the headline from the first page of the *Guidelines:* "Eating is one of life's greatest pleasures." Amen to that.

## Food and sex: What do these foods have in common?

Oysters, celery, onions, asparagus, mushrooms, truffles, chocolate, honey, caviar, bird's nest soup, and alcoholic beverages. No, that's not a menu for the very, very picky. It's a partial list of foods long reputed to be *aphrodisiacs,* substances that rev up the libido and improve sexual performance. Take a second look and you'll see why each is on the list.

Celery and asparagus are shaped something like a male sex organ. Oysters, mushrooms, and truffles are said to arouse emotion because they resemble parts of the female anatomy. Caviar (fish eggs) and bird's nest soup are symbols of fertility. Onions contain chemicals that produce a mild burning sensation when eliminated in the urine; some people, masochists to be sure, may confuse this with arousal.

Honey is the quintessential sweetener: The Bible's Song of Solomon compares it to the lips of the beloved. Alcoholic beverages relax the inhibitions (but overindulgence reduces sexual performance, especially in men). As for chocolate, well, it's a veritable lover's cocktail, with stimulants (caffeine and theobromine), a marijuana-like compound called anandamide, and phenylethylamine, a chemical produced in the bodies of people in love.

So, do these foods actually make you feel sexy? Yes and no. An aphrodisiac isn't a food that sends you in search of a lover as soon as you eat it. No, it's one that makes you feel so good that you can follow through on your natural instincts. Which is as fine a description as you're likely to get of oysters, celery, onions, asparagus, mushrooms, truffles, chocolate, honey, caviar, bird's nest soup, and wine.

# Chapter 8

# Making Wise Food Choices

················································

## In This Chapter

▶ Presenting the old and new food pyramids

▶ Using MyPyramid to tailor your diet to your age and activity level

▶ Translating the Nutrition Facts labels

▶ Putting MyPyramid and the Nutrition Facts label to work

················································

This chapter features the new Food Guide Pyramid and the Nutrition Facts labels — and it tells you how to use them to create a healthful diet.

But consider yourself warned: The following pages are packed with numbers and details, maybe more than you ever wanted to know about your daily bread — and everything else on your plate. Don't let the many, many facts and stats turn you off. The information you find here really is useful for making good food choices.

# *Playing with Blocks: Basics of the Food Pyramids*

Food pyramids are comprised of building blocks for grown-ups. Instead of letters in the alphabet, these blocks represent food groups that you can put together to create a picture of a healthful diet.

The essential message of all good guides to healthful food choices is that no one food is either good or bad — how much and how often you eat a food is what counts. With that in mind, a food pyramid delivers three important messages:

- **Variety:** The fact that the pyramid contains several blocks tells you that no single food gives you all the nutrients you need.

- **Moderation:** Having blocks smaller than others tells you that although every food is valuable, some — such as fats and sweets — are best consumed in small amounts.

- **Balance:** You can't build a pyramid with a set of identical blocks. Blocks of different sizes show that a healthful diet is balanced: the right amount from each food group.

Clearly, the virtue of a food pyramid is that using it enables you to eat practically everything you like — as long as you follow the recommendations on how much and how frequently (or infrequently) to eat it.

## *The original USDA Food Guide Pyramid*

The first food pyramid was created by the U.S. Department of Agriculture (USDA) in 1992 in response to criticism that the previous government guide to food choices — the Four Food Group Plan (vegetables and fruits, breads and cereals, milk and milk products, meat and meat alternatives) — was too heavily weighted toward high-fat, high-cholesterol foods from animals.

Figure 8-1 depicts the original USDA Food Guide Pyramid. As you can see, this pyramid is based on daily food choices, showing you which foods are in what groups. Unlike the Four Food Group Plan, the pyramid separates fruits and vegetables into two distinct groups and lists the number of servings from each food group that you should have each day. (The number of servings is provided in ranges. The lower end is for people who consume about 1,600 calories a day, and the upper end is for people whose daily dietary intake nears 3,000 calories.)

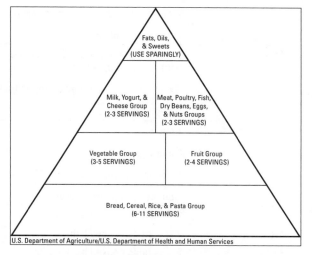

**Figure 8-1:** The original USDA Food Guide Pyramid.

How much is a serving? Not to worry. That's spelled out in Table 8-1.

| Table 8-1 | Standard Serving Sizes |
|---|---|
| *Food Group* | *Serving Size* |
| Bread | 1 slice bread |
| Cereal | 1 ounce ready-to-eat cereal |
| | ½ cup cooked cereal |
| Rice, pasta, crackers | ½ cup cooked rice or pasta |
| | 5–6 small crackers |
| Vegetables | 1 cup raw leafy vegetables |
| | ½ cup chopped raw vegetables |
| | ½ cup cooked chopped vegetables |
| | ¾ cup vegetable juice |
| Fruits | 1 medium piece of fresh fruit (apple, banana, orange, peach) |
| | ½ cup cooked or canned chopped fruit |
| | ¾ cup fruit juice |
| Milk products | 1 cup milk |
| | 1 cup yogurt |
| | 1½ ounces natural cheese |
| | 2 ounces processed cheese |
| Meat | 2–3 ounces cooked lean meat |
| Fish | 2–3 ounces cooked fish |
| Poultry | 2–3 ounces cooked lean poultry |
| Dry beans | ½ cup cooked dry beans |
| Eggs | 1 egg (1 ounce) |

| Food Group | Serving Size |
|---|---|
| Nuts, seeds | 2 tablespoons peanut butter<br>⅓ cup nuts or seeds |
| Fats, oils, sweets | No specific amount; very little |

*Source:* The Food Guide Pyramid *(Washington, D.C.: International Food Information Council Foundation, U.S. Department of Agriculture, Food Marketing Institute, 1995)*

One useful aspect of the original USDA Food Guide Pyramid is its recommendation of different numbers of daily servings for people consuming different amounts of calories each day. For example, consider how the recommended number of servings from the bread group varies at different levels of calorie consumption.

Table 8-2 lists the original USDA serving recommendations for three levels of calorie consumption:

- 1,600 calories per day (sufficient for women who don't exercise and for many older adults)

- 2,200 calories per day (meets the needs of most children, active women, and many sedentary men)

- 2,800 calories per day (provides the energy required by most teenage boys, many active men, and some very active women)

### Table 8-2 How Many Servings: Daily Choices Based on the Original USDA Food Guide Pyramid

| Food | 1,600 Calories/ Day | 2,200 Calories/ Day | 2,800 Calories/ Day |
|---|---|---|---|
| Bread group | 6 servings | 9 servings | 11 servings |
| Fruit group | 2 servings | 3 servings | 4 servings |

*(continued)*

**Table 8-2** *(continued)*

| Food | 1,600 Calories/Day | 2,200 Calories/Day | 2,800 Calories/Day |
|------|---------------------|---------------------|---------------------|
| Vegetable group | 3 servings | 4 servings | 5 servings |
| Milk group* | 2–3 servings | 2–3 servings | 2–3 servings |
| Meat group | 5 ounces | 6 ounces | 7 ounces |

* Requirements higher for women who are pregnant or nursing
Source: The Food Guide Pyramid (Washington, D.C.: International Food Information Council Foundation, U.S. Department of Agriculture, Food Marketing Institute, 1995)

## The brand-new 2005 USDA Food Guide Pyramid

By the time USDA/HHS got around to revising the *Dietary Guidelines for 2005,* it was pretty clear that the original food pyramid hadn't done its proposed job of teaching most Americans how to choose foods that provide sufficient nutrients without piling on the pounds.

What to do? What else? In a word, MyPyramid (see Figure 8-2).

Like the original Food Guide Pyramid, this new version is made up of sections representing the foods in your daily diet — from left to right, grains, vegetables, fruit, oils, milk, and meat/beans.

Like the building blocks on the original Food Guide Pyramid, the six bands on this one say "pick lots of different kinds of foods to build a better diet." The different sizes of the sections suggest that you should consume more of some foods than others. The steps going up the side of the pyramid say, "Physical activity matters, so get moving!"

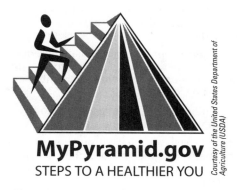

**MyPyramid.gov**
STEPS TO A HEALTHIER YOU

*Courtesy of the United States Department of Agriculture (USDA)*

**Figure 8-2:** The MyPyramid image promotes both proper diet and exercise.

And the MyPyramid slogan, "Steps to a Healthier You," tells you that you don't have to leap tall buildings in a single bound like Superman (or woman) to improve your nutrition. Even small steps can make a big difference.

But the big deal about MyPyramid is that you can personalize the diagram to meet your own special needs. For more information, visit www.mypyramid.gov.

## Understanding the Nutrition Facts Labels

Once upon a time, the only reliable consumer information on a food label was the name of the food inside. The 1990 Nutrition Labeling and Education Act changed that forever with a spiffy new set of consumer-friendly food labels that include the following:

- ✔ A mini-nutrition guide that shows the food's nutrient content and evaluates its place in a balanced diet

- ✔ Accurate ingredient listings, with all ingredients listed in order of their weight in the food — for example, the most prominent ingredient in a loaf of bread would be flour

- ✔ Clear identification of ingredients previously listed simply as *colorings* and *sweeteners*

- ✔ Scientifically reliable information about the relationship between specific foods and specific chronic health conditions, such as heart disease and cancer

The Nutrition Facts label is *required by law* for more than 90 percent of all processed, packaged foods — everything from canned soup to fresh pasteurized orange juice. Food sold in really small packages — a pack of gum, for example — can omit the nutrition label but must carry a telephone number or address so that an inquisitive consumer (you) can call or write for the information.

Just about the only processed foods exempted from the nutrition labeling regulations are those with no appreciable amounts of nutrients or those whose content varies from batch to batch:

- ✔ Plain (unflavored) coffee and tea

- ✔ Some spices and flavorings

- ✔ Deli and bakery items prepared fresh in the store where they're sold directly to the consumer, as well as food produced by small companies

- ✔ Food sold in restaurants, unless it makes a nutrition content or health claim

Labels are voluntary for fresh raw meat, fish, or poultry and fresh fruits and vegetables, but many markets — perhaps under pressure from customers (Hint! Hint!) — put posters or brochures with generic nutrition information near the meat counter or produce bins.

## *Just the facts, ma'am*

The star of the Nutrition Facts label is the Nutrition Facts panel on the back (or side) of the package. This panel features three important elements: serving sizes, amounts of nutrients per serving, and Percent Daily Value (see Figure 8-3).

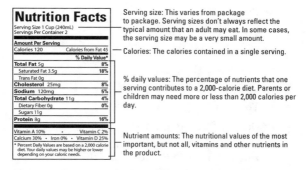

**Figure 8-3:** A typical Nutrition Facts panel.

No need to stretch your brain trying to translate gram-servings or ounce-servings into real servings. This label does it for you, listing the servings in comprehensible kitchen terms such as 1 cup or one waffle or two pieces or 1 teaspoon. It also tells you how many servings are in the package.

The serving size is exactly the same for all products in a category. In other words, the Nutrition Facts chart enables you to compare at a glance the nutrient content for two different brands of yogurt, cheddar cheese, string beans, soft drinks, and so on.

When checking the labels, you may think the suggested serving sizes seem small (especially with so-called low-fat items). Think of these serving sizes as useful guides.

The Nutrition Facts chart also tells you the amount (per serving) for several important factors:

- Calories
- Calories from fat
- Total fat (in grams)
- Saturated fat (in grams)
- Trans fats (in grams)
- Cholesterol (in milligrams)
- Total carbohydrate (in grams)
- Dietary fiber (in grams)
- Sugars (in grams — total sugars, the ones occurring naturally in the food *and* the ones added during preparation)
- Protein (in grams)

Finally, the Percent Daily Value enables you to judge whether a specific food is high, medium, or low in fat, cholesterol, sodium, carbohydrates, dietary fiber, sugar, protein, vitamin A, vitamin C, calcium, and iron.

The Percent Daily Value for vitamins and minerals is based on a set of recommendations called the *Reference Daily Intakes* (RDI), which are similar (but not identical) to the Recommended Dietary Allowances (RDAs) for vitamins and minerals.

RDIs are based on allowances set in 1973, so some RDIs now may not apply to all groups of people. For example, the Daily Value for calcium is 1,000 milligrams, but many studies — and two National Institutes of Health Conferences — suggest that post-menopausal women who are not using hormone replacement therapy need to consume 1,500 milligrams of calcium a day to reduce their risk of osteoporosis.

The Percent Daily Values for fats, carbohydrates, protein, sodium, and potassium are based on the *Daily Reference Values* (DRVs). DRVs are standards for nutrients, such as fat and fiber, known to raise or lower the risk of certain health conditions, such as heart disease and cancer. For example, the *Dietary Guidelines for Americans 2005* says that no more than 30 percent of your daily calories should come from fat. That means a 2,000-calorie-per-day diet shouldn't have any more than 600 calories from fat. To translate fat calories to grams of fat (the units used in the DRVs), divide the number of calories from fat (600) by 9 (the number of calories in one gram of fat). The answer, 67, is slightly higher than the actual DRV. But it's close enough.

Nutritionists use similar calculations to set the DRVs, such as

- ✔ Saturated fat — 10 percent of your calories/9 calories per gram

- ✔ Carbohydrates — 60 percent of your calories/4 calories per gram

- ✔ Dietary fiber — 11.5 percent of your calories/0 calories per gram

- ✔ Protein — 10 percent of your calories/4 calories per gram

Having set down this tidy list, I'm now compelled to tell you that the %DV (that's short for Percent Daily Value), as shown on the Nutrition Facts labels, are behind the times. New recommendations in the *Dietary Guidelines for Americans 2005* say

- ✔ Total fat calories should account for 20 percent to 35 percent of total daily calories.

- ✔ No safe level exists for saturated fats or trans fats, thus no %DV is provided for either one. *Note:* The total amount of saturated fat in the portion is the number of grams of saturated fat plus the number of grams of trans fat. (Who else would tell you these things?)

- ✔ Calories from carbs should account for 45 percent to 65 percent of daily calories.

- ✔ Women younger than 50 need to consume 25 grams of dietary fiber a day; men younger than 50, 38 grams. After age 51, it's 21 grams for women and 30 grams for men.

- ✔ Calories from protein should account for 10 percent to 35 percent of total daily calories, an amount much higher than the current RDA for protein.

# Organic: The not-quite-finished evolution of a label term

*Organic* (as in organic food) is a highly charged food word. But do you know what it means? Don't be embarrassed to say no. Until recently, neither did most health professionals.

To a chemist, *organic* means a substance that contains carbon, hydrogen, and oxygen. By this chemical standard, all foods — and all human beings — are organic.

Yet some people adopted the word *organic* to describe plant foods grown without pesticides or synthetic chemicals, or to describe the poultry, fish, beef, and lamb from animals raised on a diet with no antibiotics or other medicating chemicals to assure healthy and efficiently producing animals.

But these descriptions were not standards regulated by any federal agency. So USDA set out to create regulations that legally define the term:

✔ In December 1997, the USDA released its first proposal on new standards for organic foods.

✔ In May 1998, after receiving more than 280,000 comments from the public, food growers, and food marketers, the agency announced that although bioengineered and irradiated foods are safe, they're not permitted to carry the organic label.

✔ In October 1998, the USDA issued three more proposals on how animals yielding organic food are to be treated and how the agency will certify producers of organic foods.

✔ In October 2002, the USDA implemented rules saying that foods carrying the organic label must be grown without pesticides or raised without non-organic feed.

*(continued)*

*(continued)*

Sounds simple, sounds good. Sounds . . . not quite final. Barely four months later, in February 2003, Congress passed legislation allowing organic livestock to be given non-organic feed at any time the price of organic feed reaches two times that of the regular stuff. As I write this book, the whole darn thing is in a state of flux. For the latest, check your local newspaper or visit www.usda.gov to see what you can dig up. Then, dig in. Maybe.

Will this change the numbers on the Nutrition Facts labels? The sensible answer is, sure it will . . . eventually. Are the current Nutrition Facts labels still useful? Absolutely.

## Listing what's inside

The extra added attraction on the Nutrition Facts label is the complete ingredient listing, in which every single ingredient is listed in order of its weight in the product, heaviest first, lightest last. In addition, the label must spell out the true identity of some classes of ingredients known to cause allergic reactions:

- ✔ Vegetable proteins (*hydrolyzed corn protein* rather than the old-fashioned *hydrolyzed vegetable protein*)

- ✔ Milk products (*nondairy* products such as coffee whiteners may contain the milk protein caseinate, which comes from milk)

- ✔ FD&C yellow no. 5, a full, formal chemical name instead of *coloring*

Naming the precise source of sweeteners (*corn sugar monohydrate* rather than just *sugar monohydrate*) is still voluntary, but as is true of information about raw meat, fish, and poultry, manufacturers and stores just may respond to consumer pressure. (Repeat advice: Hint! Hint!)

# Choosing Foods with MyPyramid and the Nutrition Facts Label

The Food Guide Pyramid helps balance meals and snacks. In the kitchen, you can increase the nutritional value by thinking of individual dishes as mini food pyramids. At snack time, you can use the Food Guide Pyramid to choose munchies that are a valuable part of your overall daily diet.

For example, although you know that fruits and veggies are good snacks, that doesn't mean that you're stuck with boring carrot sticks or an apple. The food pyramid says "fruits and vegetables," not raw fruits and raw vegetables. Yes, a fresh apple is fine. But so is a baked apple (100 calories), fragrant with cinnamon and decorated with no-fat sour cream (30 to 45 calories for 2 tablespoons). Carrot strips are okay. So are vegetarian baked beans — yes, baked beans (140 calories plus 26 grams of carbohydrates, 7 grams of protein, 7 grams of dietary fiber, and 2 grams of fat per ½-cup serving), which are considered both veggies *and* a member of the high-protein meat/beans group.

As for the Nutrition Facts label, you can use that to eat your cake and have it nutritiously by comparing products to choose the best alternatives.

Here's a good example: You find yourself irresistibly drawn to double dark chocolate ice cream (lots of fat, saturated fat, cholesterol, and a whopping 230 calories per ½-cup serving). But then, just as your hand is opening the freezer door, ready to reach for the ice cream, suddenly . . . out of the corner of your eye, you see the Nutrition Facts panel on the label of the no-fat but equally irresistible chocolate sorbet. It says, "No fat, no saturated fat, no cholesterol, and only 90 to 130 calories per serving." When you put the labels side-by-side, do you need to ask which one comes out the winner?

# The Final Word on Diagrams and Stats

At the beginning of this chapter, I warned you that keeping track of all the facts may be difficult. But now I think that you can pretty much boil them all down to one nutritional Golden Rule exemplified by the food pyramids and the Nutrition Facts food label: *Keep things in proportion.*

Come to think of it, that's not a bad philosophy for life.

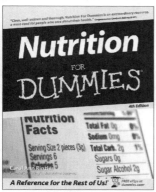
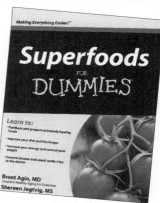
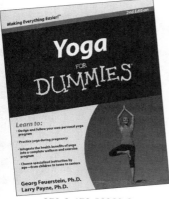
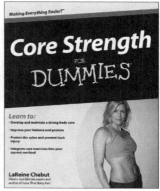

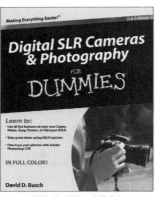
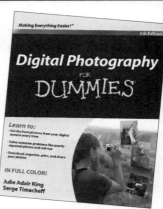
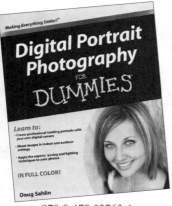
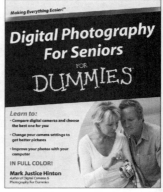

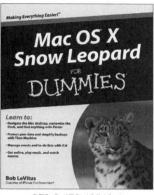
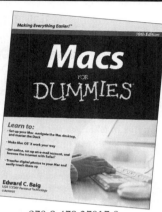
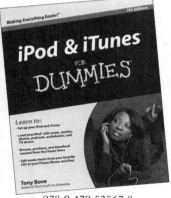
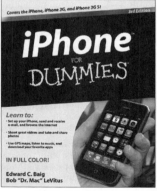

After you've read the Portable Edition, look for the original Dummies book on the topic. The handy Contents at a Glance below highlights the information you'll get when you purchase a copy of *Nutrition For Dummies*, 4th Edition — available wherever books are sold, or visit dummies.com.

# Contents at a Glance

*Introduction* .................................................................................. 1

*Part I: The Basic Facts about Nutrition* ...................................... 7
    Chapter 1: What's Nutrition, Anyway? ................................................ 9
    Chapter 2: Digestion: The 24-Hour Food Factory ............................ 19
    Chapter 3: Calories: The Energizers ................................................... 29
    Chapter 4: How Much Nutrition Do You Need? ................................ 45
    Chapter 5: A Supplemental Story ....................................................... 55

*Part II: What You Get from Food* ............................................... 67
    Chapter 6: Powerful Protein ................................................................ 69
    Chapter 7: The Lowdown on Fat and Cholesterol ............................ 81
    Chapter 8: Carbohydrates: A Complex Story ................................... 97
    Chapter 9: Alcohol: Another Form of Grape and Grain ................. 113
    Chapter 10: Vigorous Vitamins ......................................................... 125
    Chapter 11: Mighty Minerals ............................................................. 149
    Chapter 12: Phabulous Phytochemicals ......................................... 169
    Chapter 13: Water Works ................................................................... 175

*Part III: Healthy Eating* .......................................................... 185
    Chapter 14: Why You Eat When You Eat ......................................... 187
    Chapter 15: Why You Like the Foods You Like ............................... 197
    Chapter 16: What Is a Healthful Diet? .............................................. 209
    Chapter 17: Making Wise Food Choices ........................................... 221
    Chapter 18: Eating Smart When Eating Out .................................... 237

*Part IV: Food Processing* ......................................................... 247
    Chapter 19: What Is Food Processing? ............................................. 249
    Chapter 20: Cooking and Nutrition .................................................. 261
    Chapter 21: What Happens When Food Is
      Frozen, Canned, Dried, or Zapped ................................................ 279
    Chapter 22: Better Eating through Chemistry ................................ 289

*Part V: Food and Medicine* ....................................................... 299
    Chapter 23: When Food Gives You Hives ....................................... 301
    Chapter 24: Food and Mood .............................................................. 309
    Chapter 25: Food and Drug Interactions ......................................... 317
    Chapter 26: Using Food as Medicine ............................................... 325

*Part VI: The Part of Tens* ......................................................... 335
    Chapter 27: Ten Nutrition Web Sites ............................................... 337
    Chapter 28: Ten (Well, Okay, Twelve) Superstar Foods ................. 345
    Chapter 29: Ten Easy Ways to Cut Calories ................................... 355

*Index* ....................................................................................... 359